University and Public Behavioral Health

Organization Collaboration

University and Public Behavioral Health Organization Collaboration

Models for Success in Justice Contexts

**EDITED BY KIRK HEILBRUN,
H. JEAN WRIGHT II, CHRISTY GIALLELLA,
AND DAVID DEMATTEO**

OXFORD
UNIVERSITY PRESS

Oxford University Press is a department of the University of Oxford. It furthers
the University's objective of excellence in research, scholarship, and education
by publishing worldwide. Oxford is a registered trade mark of Oxford University
Press in the UK and certain other countries.

Published in the United States of America by Oxford University Press
198 Madison Avenue, New York, NY 10016, United States of America.

© Oxford University Press 2021

All rights reserved. No part of this publication may be reproduced, stored in
a retrieval system, or transmitted, in any form or by any means, without the
prior permission in writing of Oxford University Press, or as expressly permitted
by law, by license, or under terms agreed with the appropriate reproduction
rights organization. Inquiries concerning reproduction outside the scope of the
above should be sent to the Rights Department, Oxford University Press, at the
address above.

You must not circulate this work in any other form
and you must impose this same condition on any acquirer.

Library of Congress Control Number: 2020057170
ISBN 978–0–19–005285–0

DOI: 10.1093/med/9780190052850.001.0001

9 8 7 6 5 4 3 2 1

Printed by Marquis, Canada

CONTENTS

This book is about collaboration. In particular, it focuses on the collaboration between universities and public behavioral health agencies and the work they do together in providing services, influencing policy, and conducting research relevant to individuals who are involved in the legal system. The idea for this volume grew out of our respective interests in these areas—and in how the work might be done better through this kind of collaboration.

The volume includes nine examples of collaborative projects: eight in the United States and one in Australia. We are grateful to the contributors who have described each. We also would like to thank our advisory board (Joel Dvoskin, Raymond Patterson, and Janet Warren) for their valuable assistance. The projects described in this book are quite varied, and while they are not necessarily representative of this kind of collaboration more broadly, they do share one common feature: they have been successful. Considering this success and the project variables associated with it has been an important goal for us.

This work was started well before the onset of COVID-19 and is being completed in the midst of a global pandemic. We can't anticipate how this pandemic will ultimately affect the kind of work that is described in these chapters, of course. But if adaptiveness, mutual respect, and "working smart" (all features of successful collaborations) remain important in the years to come, then these successful collaborations may be particularly relevant in our path forward.

—Kirk Heilbrun, H. Jean Wright II, Christy Giallella,
and David DeMatteo
Philadelphia, Pennsylvania
May 2020

CONTRIBUTORS

David Ayers
Department of Behavioral Health and
 Justice Related Services
Philadelphia Department of
 Behavioral Health and Intellectual
 disAbility Services
Chalfont, PA, USA

Joshua T. Barnett, MHS, MA
Department of Mental Health Law
 and Policy
University of South Florida
Sarasota, FL, USA

Natalie Bonfine, PhD
Department of Psychiatry
Northeast Ohio Medical University
Rootstown, OH, USA

Richard J. Bonnie, JD
Schools of Law, Medicine, and
 Public Policy
University of Virginia
Charlottesville, VA, USA

Melissa Carlson, BS
Department of Mental Health Law
 and Policy
University of South Florida
Tampa, FL, USA

Annette Christy, PhD
Department of Mental Health Law
 and Policy
University of South Florida
Tampa, FL, USA

Mary Alice Conroy, PhD, ABPP
Department of Psychology
Sam Houston State University
Huntsville, TX, USA

David DeMatteo, JD, PhD
Department of Psychology and
 Thomas R. Kline School of Law
Drexel University
Blue Bell, PA, USA

Alisha Desai, MS
Department of Psychology
Drexel University
Denver, CO, USA

Kelley Durham, MS
Department of Psychology
Drexel University
Madison, CT, USA

Elizabeth Gale-Bentz, PhD
Health Services Division
Harris County Juvenile Probation
 Department
Houston, TX, USA

Christy Giallella, PhD
Department of Behavioral Health and
  Justice Related Services
Philadelphia Department of
  Behavioral Health and Intellectual
  disAbility Services
Burlington, NJ, USA

Naomi E. Goldstein, PhD
Department of Psychology
Drexel University
Philadelphia, PA, USA

Patricia Griffin, PhD
Wyndmoor, PA, USA

Thomas Grisso, PhD
Department of Psychiatry
University of Massachusetts
  Medical School
Shrewsbury, MA, USA

Kirk Heilbrun, PhD
Department of Psychology
Drexel University
Philadelphia, PA, USA

Rena Kreimer, MSW
Department of Psychology
Drexel University
Philadelphia, PA, USA

Claire Lankford, MS
Department of Psychology
Drexel University
Alexander City, AL, USA

Benjamin Locklair, JD, PhD
Behavioral Health and Justice Related
  Services
Philadelphia Department of
  Behavioral Health and Intellectual
  Disabilities
Philadelphia, PA, USA

Barbara McDermott, PhD
Department of Psychiatry and
  Behavioral Sciences
University of California, Davis
Sacramento, CA, USA

Jeanne McPhee, MS
Department of Psychology
Drexel University
Philadelphia, PA, USA

Marie McPherson, MBA
Department of Mental Health Law
  and Policy
University of South Florida
Tampa, FL, USA

Kathleen Moore, PhD
Louis de la Parte Florida Mental
  Health Institute
College of Behavioral and
  Community Sciences,
  Department of Mental
  Health Law and Policy
Tampa, FL, USA

Mark R. Munetz, MD
Department of Psychiatry
Northeast Ohio Medical University
Rootstown, OH, USA

Daniel C. Murrie, PhD
Institute of Law, Psychiatry, and
  Public Policy
University of Virginia School of
  Medicine
Charlottesville, VA, USA

Christopher Nicastro, MA, LPCC
Ohio Department of Mental Health
  and Addiction Services
Powell, OH, USA

James R. P. Ogloff, BA, MA, JD, PhD
Centre for Forensic Behavioural
  Science
Swinburne University of Technology
  and Forensicare
Alphington, VIC, Australia

Ira K. Packer, PhD, ABPP (Forensic)
Department of Psychiatry
University of Massachusetts
  Medical School
Worcester, MA, USA

Victoria Pietruszka, MS, JD
Department of Psychology
Drexel University
Uxbridge, MA, USA

Rosa Viñas Racionero, PhD
University of Nebraska Public
    Policy Center
Lincoln, NE, USA

Mario J. Scalora, PhD
Department of Psychology
University of Nebraska-Lincoln
Lincoln, NE, USA

Charles Scott, MD
Department of Psychiatry and
    Behavioral Sciences
University of California, Davis
Sacramento, CA, USA

Ruth H. Simera, MEd, LSW
Department of Psychiatry
Northeast Ohio Medical University
Garrettsville, OH, USA

Katherine Warburton, DO
CA Department of State Hospitals
Napa, CA, USA

H. Jean Wright II, PsyD
Department of Psychology
Temple University
Philadelphia, PA, USA

Heather Zelle, JD, PhD
Institute of Law, Psychiatry, and
    Public Policy
University of Virginia
Charlottesville, VA, USA

Kirk Heilbrun is currently a Professor in the Department of Psychology at Drexel University, where he served as department head from 1999–2012 and 2014–2016. He is board certified in clinical psychology and in forensic psychology by the American Board of Professional Psychology, and is a Fellow of the American Psychological Association in six divisions. He currently directs a forensic assessment clinic in the Drexel Department of Psychology and the Reentry Project, another Drexel-based project that provides pro bono assessment and treatment services to justice-involved individuals returning to the community from federal prison or under the jurisdiction of the federal mental health court.

H. Jean Wright II is an Adjunct Professor in the Department of Psychology at Temple University. Dr. Wright previously served as Clinical Director of the Juvenile Justice initiative, within the Philadelphia Behavioral Health System, and is the former Program Director for the city's Mental Health First Aid (MHFA) initiative. He also spends considerable time conducting seminars, workshops, and trainings on a variety of topics related to behavioral health and wellness, public health education, and trauma-informed care, for a diverse group of clientele.

Christy Giallella is the Clinical Forensic Manager with Behavioral Health and Justice Related Services of the Philadelphia Department of Behavioral Health and Intellectual disAbility Services. Her work seeks to improve policies and programs for justice-involved individuals with behavioral health challenges. Dr. Giallella earned her PhD in Clinical Psychology from Drexel University. She is a licensed clinical psychologist with a specialization in forensic psychology. Dr. Giallella has worked in a variety of community-based and correctional settings with justice-involved adolescents and adults, conducting assessments and providing treatment. Her research background includes juvenile justice, forensic mental health assessment, and public policy.

David DeMatteo is a Professor of Psychology and Law at Drexel University, and Director of Drexel's JD/PhD Program in Law and Psychology. His research interests include offender diversion, psychopathic personality, and forensic mental health assessment, and his research has been funded by several federal agencies, state agencies, and private foundations. He is a Fellow of the American Psychological Association (Divisions 12 and 41), a Fellow of the American Academy of Forensic Psychology, and board certified in forensic psychology by the American Board of Professional Psychology. He is also a former President of the American Psychology-Law Society (APA Division 41).

Introduction

KIRK HEILBRUN, H. JEAN WRIGHT II, CHRISTY GIALLELLA,
DAVID DEMATTEO, KELLEY DURHAM,
AND CLAIRE LANKFORD ■

There are various influences on the contemporary delivery of behavioral health services to individuals involved in the criminal justice system. One involves the findings from empirical research. From drug trials to psychotherapy research, from the development of relevant psychological tests and specialized measures to the most effective approach to providing reentry services, there are many services that are guided by translational research. Yet the time and specialization to conduct and consider such translational research are often limited by the service demands on public behavioral health organizations (PBHOs) that provide assessment and intervention to justice-involved individuals. Accordingly, collaboration with university-based specialists that would promote empirically guided practice and decision-making could be sensible and practical.

There are additional justifications for university–PBHO collaboration that go beyond the more efficient use of research and other resources. Grant funding agencies, faced with their own shrinking budgets, are more inclined to fund projects that include large samples and provide interventions that can demonstrate immediate impact. PBHOs can often provide access to the individuals and contexts that enhance the value of grant-funded research, adding appeal to a partnership with applied researchers in academic settings. Universities also train the next generation of practitioners, clinical leaders, and applied researchers. There can be strong training value to supervised experience with PBHOs, particularly for trainees interested in policy as well as practice. As part of such supervised experience, trainees themselves can also provide valuable service contributions.

There can also be significant advantages to PBHOs that accrue from such partnerships. The quality of services provided by PBHOs may be enhanced through greater access to research findings available in the national literature. They may also be improved through evaluating the effectiveness of their own programming, which can be assisted by university-based collaborators. More generally, the diversity of perspectives available through such partnerships can enhance the quality of decision-making and problem-solving. In addition, some PBHOs may recruit more effectively to fill available staff positions when university-based trainees are part of the collaboration. The training of such individuals can also be improved when they have access to relevant experience provided by PBHOs.

This book's major purpose is to offer detailed information about successful university–PBHO collaboration. The various chapters provide different examples of such collaborations. These examples were selected by their reputations for success. We did not have a systematic empirical basis for such selections, but there was strong anecdotal evidence that each of these collaborations is well-operated and has provided valued services.

The chapter authors offer detailed descriptions of their respective collaborations. These descriptions cover various aspects of the collaboration, including purposes, beginning, leadership, who is served, services, operations, effectiveness measurement, financial arrangements, and lessons learned. This chapter and the last chapter are provided by the editors, offering context and analysis, respectively, for those who participate in a university–PBHO collaboration—or might be interested in doing so.

RELEVANT TERMS AND CONSTRUCTS

It is important to be clear about the organizations, contexts, and outcomes that will be described in this book. We offer five definitions in this section.

University: This will be defined as an advanced educational organization of any size. It may be either public or private.

Public behavioral health organization: This is a public, non-university entity that delivers behavioral health services (including assessment and intervention to individuals with problems in domains including mental health, substance abuse, and cognitive or intellectual disability). At least some of these services are provided to justice-involved individuals.

Criminal justice involvement: This refers to involvement with public safety officers, specialized (problem-solving) and traditional courts, court clinics, prosecution and defense attorneys, correctional facilities (jails and prisons), and/or parole and probation. The contact may be informal, involving questioning that does not lead to arrest. It may also be formal but include diversion from the traditional path of prosecution, conviction, and incarceration or community supervision. Finally, it may involve the traditional path, with individuals going through reentry following incarceration and release to the community.

Collaboration: This is a formal agreement with several components. There is a contract (oral or written), a designated period of collaboration, and specified services—and remuneration for such services.

Judgments about meaningful outcomes: There are several ways in which we will consider how meaning is assigned to outcomes. When measures are quantified, then statistical analyses of significance may be used. In combination with such statistical analyses, the collaboration may consider whether outcomes are "clinically significant"—whether they are of a nature and magnitude that reflect important differences or outcomes in that particular context. Finally, there may be judgments about meaning that are made in the absence of quantified measures, focusing more on qualitative data from key stakeholders and the recipients of services.

REVIEW OF RELEVANT LITERATURE

Several aspects of the literature in this area are apparent, as we discuss in this section. While neither extensive nor well-developed, this literature does offer some attention to university–PBHO collaborations. (This is often presented in terms such as "researcher–practitioner" collaboration.) There are two empirical studies and one special issue of a journal, but the remainder of the articles represent the perspectives of a single discussant, team, or jurisdiction. There is no obvious pattern to be seen in who constitutes the "practitioner" partner in the collaboration; among those represented are the criminal justice system generally, police, departments of corrections, juvenile agencies, problem-solving courts, and departments of parole and probation.

Empirical Survey

The most substantial empirical study (Sullivan, Willie, & Fisher, 2013) involved a grant-funded investigation of researcher–practitioner collaborations in the United States and Canada, with the goal of identifying the "highlights" and "lowlights" of such collaborations. There were two components to this study. First, individual interviews and focus groups were conducted with researchers and practitioners who reported having at least one "successful" research partnership. "Practitioners" were those employed by criminal justice state administrative agencies or those who provided services to justice-involved clients. "Researchers" were not employees of the criminal justice system. Participants included 55 women and 17 men of various racial/ethnic groups, employed in urban, suburban, and rural settings in the United States and Canada, including family violence and sexual assault programs, private practice, and administrative agencies such as departments of corrections, local county courts, independent research institutes, and colleges/universities. Interviews were conducted with 49 people (38 women and 11 men). Focus group participation was facilitated for 23 participants (17 women and 6 men) in five groups, held at professional conferences. Data analysis was both qualitative and quantitative, focusing on the following aspects of the collaboration: highlights, lowlights, reasons it was needed, benefits, desirable aspects of collaborators and organizations, facilitation of success, challenges to success, balancing needs of researchers and participants, products and their usefulness, sustainability, and advice for both researchers and practitioners.

Second, a survey of state administrative agencies was conducted to describe each state's infrastructure and general experiences regarding research in the criminal justice system, and document lessons learned from successful collaborations with outside researchers. Participants were those responsible for overseeing agency research or conducting it on behalf of the agency; they were employed by the agency. A total of 75 participants from 49 states completed the survey. A total of 41% were administrators or directors of the agency, 35% were supervisors or managers, and 21% were front-line or support staff.

The following were described as highlights of such collaboration:

- A strong relationship between the researcher and practitioner was key.
- The researcher was knowledgeable about the system and "walked in the shoes" of the practitioner.
- Practitioners learned the basics of conducting research.
- The project was developed and carried out in a truly collaborative manner.
- Administrators were invested and helped move the project forward.
- Findings had direct relevance to services and policies for practitioners and clients.

The more problematic aspects of collaboration ("lowlights") were identified as well:

- Collaborations took longer than projects done by a researcher alone— and longer than practitioners imagined.
- Past negative experiences or misunderstandings about researchers and the research process contributed to a distrust of researchers by practitioners.
- High staff turnover contributed to difficulties in keeping staff invested and completing projects.

Journal Special Issue

A special issue of *Criminal Justice Studies* (volume 27, 2014) focused on developing and sustaining collaborative research partnerships between universities and criminal justice agencies. Noting that there had been little attention paid to this topic in scholarly journals, the special edition editors (Childs & Potter, 2014) observed that such partnerships are seen in public health, business, medicine, and the social sciences. These editors also noted that there are distinguishing aspects to criminal justice partnerships, such as data sensitivity, available funding, and the large number of agencies involved in a single project.

Three of the articles in this special issue focused on collaboration in the general context of the criminal justice system rather than in one specific area. In the first (Nilson, Jewell, Camman, Appell, & Wormith, 2014), the authors described their academic research center focused on community-engaged scholarship with criminal justice partners from government and nonprofit sectors. They address the topics of research relevance, outcome measurement, data collection methods, expectations, communication, and organizational change. They also incorporate the perspectives of their collaborative justice partners: these included capacity building, program improvement, and decision-making. Among the "key ingredients" for successful partnerships were continuous communication, formalization of the partnership, and clear expectations regarding expected deliverables.

The second article with a broad focus on collaboration (Rudes, Viglione, Lerch, Porter, & Taxman, 2014) identified relevant components including access, agreement, goal setting, feedback, and relationship maintenance. They illustrated the successful collaboration process by describing four partnerships between a specialized center for correctional excellence and various criminal justice agencies (including probation and parole and problem-solving courts) at the federal, state, and county levels.

Drawing on their experience in Syracuse, New York, the authors of the third article (Worden, McLean, & Bonner, 2014) offered a description of various partnerships over a 20-year period between academics and practitioners. They identified sustainability as a major challenge to using such research partnerships in a maximally effective way. Factors supporting success—and those challenging it—were identified. Like the first two articles, this one was reasonably optimistic about the prospect of developing and operating partnerships but less optimistic about sustaining any particular collaboration for a substantial time. This may reflect the reality that some partnerships are developed to address a fairly specific set of problems and are no longer needed when those problems have been addressed.

The fourth relevant article in this special issue focused on a partnership between university researchers and federal probation (Clodfelter, Alexander, Holcomb, Marcum, & Richards, 2014). It was specific not only in identifying a particular criminal justice agency, but also a designated purpose: the assessment of an ongoing training program to improve officer interactions with offenders. This may illustrate our point in the previous paragraph. When a collaboration is developed for a very specific reason, there may be a built-in shelf life—particularly if university researchers provide the practitioner partner with the tools to continue an ongoing program evaluation once the structure of this evaluation has been established.

Epidemiology

In covering this topic (Buckeridge et al., 2002), university researchers in Canada describe a collaboration with community health officials to improve access to community health information. Project objectives included (1) the development of a geographic information system to access routinely collected health data and to consider various problems encountered during system development and (2) the analysis of challenges encountered in the process of this collaboration. They identified several important influences on the success of this joint effort. These included the differences between community and university cultures, time constraints, and the impact of uncertainty and ambiguity on the collaborative process.

Police

Three articles have addressed collaboration between universities and police. In the first (Burkhardt et al., 2017), the focus was on the problem involving a substantial increase in the number of contacts between police and community members showing symptoms of mental illness. This initial question resulted in a collaborative consideration of the nature, causes, and consequences of this increase. Describing the collaboration from the perspectives of both police and university investigators, the authors drew on their experience with this and previous collaborations to discuss benefits, challenges, and recommendations for university–police research collaborations. Among the challenges identified were relationship definition, data collection and analysis, products, and relationship maintenance. They concluded, however, that the potential benefits for both researchers and law enforcement agencies are considerable.

Another article focusing on collaborations with police (Guillaume, Sidebottom, & Tilley, 2012) describes the experience of an extended collaborative relationship in Great Britain between a specialized university institute (UCL Jill Dando Institute of Security and Crime Science at University College London) and Warwickshire Police. This is another example of a very specific problem for collaboration: reducing bag theft from British supermarkets. It also provides another example of a collaboration being facilitated by the a priori existence of a specialized institute focusing on the particular kind of problem that is of interest to a community agency.

Finally, a third article (Rojek, Smith, & Alpert, 2012) described the findings from a national survey of law enforcement agencies on research partnership participation. This survey strongly suggests that publications in scholarly and professional journals reflect only a small portion of the ongoing collaborations between researchers and practitioners because it indicated that almost one-third of responding police agencies had participated in a research partnership within the past 5 years. Other respondents noted that they did not have funding to do so—but perhaps would have participated if such funding had been available.

Departments of Corrections

There are several relevant articles describing collaborative partnerships between university researchers and correctional agencies. Earlier work (Welsh, 2000) described several services provided by a specialized center at Temple University, in Philadelphia, and the state department of corrections. Such services included a descriptive assessment of drug and alcohol programming, an evaluation of drug and alcohol programs at two correctional facilities, and the development of an outcome evaluation research design. In addition to these services, an important outcome involved developing a working research relationship between the university and the department of corrections. The collaboration eventually produced a database of 118 prison-based drug and alcohol treatment programs at different correctional facilities, reflecting considerable variability in program duration and intensity but more consistency in treatment approach and criteria for treatment completion. It also yielded a successful research partnership with positive mutual feedback and a continuing relationship with an active research agenda. The evaluation of the prison-based drug treatment was eventually grant-funded, with the project described in a final report (Welsh, 2002).

Another article from the *Criminal Justice Studies* special issue described the partnership between Florida State University and the Florida Department of Corrections (Bales, Scaggs, Clark, Ensley, & Coltharp, 2014). It addressed the origin, development, challenges, and value (both short- and long-term) of this partnership. Its development and successful maintenance was facilitated by a grant from the National Institute of Justice, underscoring the value of extramural funding at some stage of the collaboration.

A subsequent description of another university–corrections department partnership (Drawbridge, Taheri, & Frost, 2018) suggests that both academic and practitioner partners are enriched by this kind of collaboration. Researchers benefit from developing better-informed questions, while practitioners can develop a better appreciation for how research can be applied to improving services. The benefits and challenges to partnerships and recommendations for building and sustaining researcher–practitioner partnerships were discussed, as illustrated by this particular collaboration.

A recent empirical study (Pesta, Blomberg, Ramos, & Ranson, 2019) reviewed two researcher–practitioner partnerships and conducted interviews with 20 researchers, policy-makers, and state-level decision-makers in correctional agencies in Florida. Of particular interest is their identification of common barriers and facilitators that affect the use of research in practice of criminal and juvenile justice. Frequently cited barriers included research being difficult to use, unsupportive leadership, ideology and politics, differential training, poor relationships, budget concerns, crisis-driven events, and time constraints. Facilitating influences included successful relationships, supportive leadership, informative research, budget concerns, and cross training. Participants stressed the value of trust, building relationships over time, communication, using data to collaborate, and genuinely understanding the goals and methods of their partners.

Juvenile Interventions

Another article (Bumbarger & Campbell, 2012) describes a decade-long collaborative relationship between the Prevention Research Center at Pennsylvania State University and the Pennsylvania Commission on Crime and Delinquency. This partnership evolved into a multiagency initiative supporting the implementation of evidence-based prevention and intervention programs and documenting their impact through a series of studies reflecting a significant and sustained impact on youth outcomes and more efficient use of system resources. The authors describe how the collaboration developed into a broader prevention-oriented infrastructure and discuss the partnership in terms of "lessons learned." It is noteworthy that the Pennsylvania Commission on Crime and Delinquency is not a service delivery agency but is instead charged with providing state-level grants and contracts to agencies that do provide such services. This is a somewhat different model, with a specialized university center working closely with a funding agency, and has implications for how funding would be obtained and the products that would be expected in exchange.

PLAN FOR THE VOLUME

This volume includes 11 chapters. In this chapter, we provide an overview of collaborative relationships between universities and PBHOs in criminal justice-related contexts. This includes a rationale for focusing on this topic, a definition of relevant constructs to be included, and a review of the existing literature in this area.

The next nine chapters are invited contributions from individuals who have been involved in this kind of collaborative relationship. Authors were asked to address a number of questions:

- *Purpose of the collaboration*: Why was the relationship initiated? There may have been very specific reasons supported by careful justifications provided in writing and reviewed at multiple levels. Alternatively, the reasons may have been much less clear, the justification less extensive, and the review less multilayered. The focus may have been on specific projects or services—or more inclined toward promoting the collaboration of specific individuals.
- *When and why the collaboration began*: How would the collaborators describe the initiation of their mutual work in the context in which it began? There may have been a specific need for services or data. A certain kind of funding (e.g., a grant award, a budget enhancement) might have created a climate conducive to such collaboration. An urgent problem or crisis might have enhanced the need for research or service as well. Whatever the purpose and circumstances associated with the initiation of the collaboration, their description will be valuable in understanding this particular work as well as useful in identifying recurring patterns across collaborations.
- *The process involved in setting it up*: This question traces the evolution of the collaboration from its initiation to the time at which it is more mature. How would the details of the collaboration's development

be described? If it involved a transition from a prior project, what steps were taken to move from the prior project to the collaboration? Chapter authors are asked to identify key contributions to the setup stage.

- *Who is involved, including leadership*: One important aspect of any collaboration involves the number of individuals involved and the approximate time commitment of these individuals. In addition, it is useful to know how the collaboration is led. There is likely to be some sharing of leadership responsibilities given that two organizations are working together. How does this work?
- *What services are delivered*: There are numerous kinds of services that could be delivered as part of this kind of collaboration. These include training, supervision, clinical services, research services, and program evaluation. The nature of the services that are provided and whether there is some combination of services are important aspects of the collaboration that can supplement the process information obtained in the previous bullet points.
- *Who is served*: What is the target population for the receipt of the services provided as part of this collaboration? Those using such services will, of course, depend on what is provided. But there is an important distinction among agency personnel, university-based trainees providing services to the agency, and individuals who themselves receive agency services. Depending on the services provided, there may be multiple target populations.
- *How the collaboration functions*: The next important question is how the collaboration is run after it has been established. What are the details of the day-to-day operation, including leadership, communication, goal-setting, products, reviews, and evaluation of effectiveness?
- *The expectations and agreements that have worked best*: In any organizational collaboration there are areas of strength. This item will identify the authors' perceptions of the aspects of the collaboration that have worked particularly smoothly or effectively.
- *The expectations and agreements that have not worked well (including the biggest mistakes)*: In a similar vein, any collaboration will have aspects of the relationship that have not worked as well. This question will include a request to identify mistakes as well as weaknesses, which may be helpful in the eventual analysis of how a university–PBHO collaboration can avoid such mistakes.
- *The significant changes since it began*: In the evolution of a successful collaboration there will have been important changes. The nature of these changes and the reasons they were made will be sought in this section.
- *The contractual details, including financial arrangements*: It seems likely that most collaborations will have developed a formal written agreement since these collaborations, by definition, involve the delivery

of services in exchange for compensation. The detailing of such written agreements, including a description of services and compensation, will be discussed.

- *How effectiveness is measured, including monitoring, data, and outcomes*: Appraising the nature of services and their outcomes can be done in at least two ways. First, were the services delivered as anticipated? Second, were the products or outcomes that may have been associated with such services tracked? The nature of this effectiveness appraisal process will be described in this section.
- *Lessons learned, with implications for other collaborations*: One of the most valuable aspects of a successful collaboration can involve the reflection of those involved about how they have been informed by the experience, what lessons have been learned, and what implications might be identified to help inform others considering a similar collaboration. Chapter contributors were invited to draw their own conclusions about their specific collaborations. The editors considered all collaborations in the aggregate to reach broader conclusions.

The final chapter undertakes the analysis of the information provided in the immediately preceding chapters, each of which has focused on a collaboration in a single site. The analysis considers both common ground and divergent aspects of the collaborations. In some instances, we may have the benefit of empirical data that have been collected to help appraise whether significant change (clinical or statistical) has resulted from the operation of the collaboration. This information, along with the "lessons learned" provided by chapter authors, will form the basis for conclusions about starting and successfully operating a collaboration between a university and a PBHO in a criminal justice context. Recommendations for successful development and operation, including the potential costs and benefits, will follow from these conclusions.

REFERENCES

Bales, W. D,, Scaggs, S. J., Clark, C. L., Ensley, D., & Coltharp, P. (2014). Researcher practitioner partnerships: A case of the development of a long-term collaborative project between a university and a criminal justice agency. *Criminal Justice Studies, 27*, 294–307. https://doi.org/10.1080/1478601X.2014.947807

Buckeridge, D. L., Mason, R., Robertson, A., Frank, J., Glazier, R., Purdon, L., . . . Hulchanski, D. (2002). Making health data maps: A case study of a community/university research collaboration. *Social Science & Medicine, 55*, 1189–1206. https://doi.org/10.1016/S0277 9536(01)00246-5

Bumbarger, B. K., & Campbell, E. M. (2012). A state agency–university partnership for translational research and the dissemination of evidence-based prevention and intervention. *Administration and Policy in Mental Health and Mental Health Services Research, 39*, 268–277. https://doi.org/10.1007/s10488-011-0372-x

Burkhardt, B. C., Akins, S., Sassaman, J., Jackson, S., Elwer, K., Lanfear, C., . . . Stevens, K. (2017). University researcher and law enforcement collaboration: Lessons from a study of justice-involved persons with suspected mental illness. *International Journal of Offender Therapy and Comparative Criminology, 61*, 508–525. https://doi.org/10.1177/0306624X15599393

Childs, K. K., & Potter, R. H. (2014). Developing and sustaining collaborative research partnerships with universities and criminal justice agencies. *Criminal Justice Studies, 27*, 245–248. https://doi.org/10.1080/1478601X.2014.947810

Clodfelter, T. A., Alexander, M. A., Holcomb, J. E., Marcum, C. D., & Richards, T. N. (2014). Improving probation officer effectiveness through agency–university collaboration. *Criminal Justice Studies, 27*, 308–322. https://doi.org/10.1080/1478601X.2014.947811

Drawbridge, D., Taheri, S., & Frost, N. (2018). Building and sustaining academic researcher and criminal justice practitioner partnerships: A corrections example. *American Journal of Crminal Justice, 43*, 627–640.

Guillaume, P., Sidebottom, A., & Tilley, N. (2012). On police and university collaborations: A problem-oriented policing case study. *Police Practice and Research, 13*, 389–401. https://doi.org/10.1080/15614263.2012.671621

Nilson, C., Jewell, L. M., Camman, C., Appell, R., & Wormith, J. S. (2014). Community engaged scholarship: The experience of ongoing collaboration between criminal justice professionals and scholars at the University of Saskatchewan. *Criminal Justice Studies, 27*, 264–277. https://doi.org/10.1080/1478601X.2014.947809

Pesta, G. B., Blomberg, T. G., Ramos, J., & Ranson, J. A. (2019). Translational criminology: Toward best practice. *American Journal of Criminal Justice, 44*, 449–518. https://doi.org/10.1007/s12103-018-9467-1

Rojek, J., Smith, H. P., & Alpert, G. P. (2012). The prevalence and characteristics of police practitioner–researcher partnerships. *Police Quarterly, 15*, 241–261. https://doi.org/10.1177/1098611112440698

Rudes, D. S., Viglione, J., Lerch, J., Porter, C., & Taxman, F. S. (2014). Build to sustain: Collaborative partnerships between university researchers and criminal justice practitioners. *Criminal Justice Studies, 27*, 249–263. https://doi.org/10.1080/1478601X.2014.947808

Sullivan, T. P., Willie, T. C., & Fisher, B. S. (2013). Highlights and lowlights of researcher practitioner collaborations in the criminal justice system: Findings from the Researcher Practitioner Partnerships Study (RPPS). Report submitted to the US Department of Justice. www. ncjrs. gov/pdffiles1/nij/grants/243914.pdf.

Welsh, W. N. (2000). Building an effective research collaboration between the Center for Public Policy at Temple University and the Pennsylvania Department of Corrections. Philadelphia, PA: Center for Public Policy, Temple University. http://www.ncjrs.gov/App/publications/abstract.aspx?ID=197067

Worden, R. E., McLean, S. J., & Bonner, H. S. (2014). Research partners in criminal justice: Notes from Syracuse. *Criminal Justice Studies, 27*, 278–293. https://doi.org/10.1080/1478601X.2014.947812

Further Reading

Backes, B., & Rorie, M. (2013). Partners in research: Lessons learned in Los Angeles. *National Institute of Justice Journal, 272*, 47–52. https://www.ncjrs.gov/pdffiles1/nij/241925.pdf

Bevilacqua, J. J., Morris, J. A., & Pumariega, A. J. (1996). State services research capacity: Building a state infrastructure for mental health services research. *Community Mental Health Journal, 32*, 519–533. http://ezproxy2.library.drexel.edu/login?url=https://search-proquestcom.ezproxy2.library.drexel.edu/docview/78506040?accountid=10559

Bruns, E. J., Hoagwood, K. E., Rivard, J. C., Wotring, J., Marsenich, L., & Carter, B. (2008). State implementation of evidence-based practice for youths, part II: Recommendations for research and policy. *Journal of the American Academy of Child and Adolescent Psychiatry, 47*, 499–504. https://doi.org/10.1097/CHI.0b013e3181684557

Caplan, G., & Caplan, B. (1999). *Mental health consultation and collaboration: Concepts and applications.* Long Grove, IL: Waveland Press.

Carise, D., Cornely, W., & Gurel, O. (2002). A successful research-practitioner collaboration in substance abuse treatment. *Journal of Substance Abuse Treatment, 23*, 157–162. https://doi.org/10.1016/S0740- 5472(02)00260-X

Cissner, A. B., & Farole, D. J. (2009). Avoiding failures of implementation: Lessons from process evaluations. Center for Court Innovation. http://www.ncjrs.gov/App/publications/abstract.aspx?ID=241174

Corse, S. J., Hirschinger, N. B., & Caldwell, S. (1996). Conducting treatment outcome research in a community mental health center: A university–agency collaboration. *Psychiatric Rehabilitation Journal, 20*, 59–63. http://dx.doi.org/10.1037/h0095399

Gondolf, E. W. (2010). Lessons from a successful and failed random assignment testing batterer program innovations. *Journal of Experimental Criminology, 6*, 355–376. https://doi.org/10.1007/s11292-010-9104-6

Goode, J., & Lumsden, K. (2018). The McDonaldisation of police–academic partnerships: Organisational and cultural barriers encountered in moving from research on police to research with police. *Policing and Society, 28*, 75–89. https://doi.org/10.1080/10439463.2016.1147039

Harrell, A., Newmark, L., & Visher, C. (2007). *Final report on the evaluation of the judicial oversight demonstration, volume 2): Findings and lessons on implementation.* Final report for the National Institute of Justice. Washington, DC: The Urban Institute.

Harrell, A., Newmark, L., Visher, C., & Castro, J. (2007). *Final report on the evaluation of the judicial oversight demonstration, volume 1: The impact of JOD in Dorchester and Washtenaw County.* Final report for the National Institute of Justice. Washington, DC: The Urban Institute.

Jurik, N. C., Blumenthal, J., Smith, B., & Portillos, E. L. (2000). Organizational cooptation or social change? A critical perspective on community-criminal justice partnerships. *Journal of Contemporary Criminal Justice, 16*, 293–320. https://doi.org/10.1177/1043986200016003004

Lane, J., Turner, S., & Flores, C. (2004). Researcher-practitioner collaboration in community corrections: Overcoming hurdles for successful partnerships. *Criminal Justice Review, 29*, 97–114. https://doi. org/10.1177/073401680402900107

Latessa, E. (2004). The challenge of change: Correction programs and evidence-based practices. *Criminology & Public Policy*, 3, 547–560. https://doi.org/10.1111/j.1745 9133.2004.tb00061.x

McFarland, B. H., DiBlasio, F. A., & Belcher, J. R. (1993). Collaborative research in mental health. *Administration and Policy in Mental Health, 20*, 421–435. https://doi.org/10.1007/BF00706287

Spohn, C., & Tellis, K. (2012). Policing and prosecuting sexual assault in Los Angeles city and county: A collaborative study in partnership with the Los Angeles Police Department, the Los Angeles County Sheriff's Department, and the Los Angeles County District Attorney's Office. Washington, DC: US Department of Justice, National Institute of Justice NCJ, 237582. https://www.ncjrs.gov/pdffiles1/nij/grants/237582.pdf

Sullivan, T. P., Price, C., McPartland, T., Hunter, B. A., & Fisher, B. S. (2017). The Researcher Practitioner Partnership Study (RPPS): Experiences from criminal justice system collaborations studying violence against women. *Violence Against Women, 23*, 887–907. https://doi.org/10.1177/1077801216650290

Talbott, J., & Robinowitz, C. (1986). *Working together: State–university collaboration in mental health (issues in psychiatry)*. Washington, DC: American Psychiatric Association.

Tillyer, R., Tillyer, M. S., McCluskey, J., Cancino, J., Todaro, J., & McKinnon, L. (2014). Researcher–practitioner partnerships and crime analysis: A case study in action research. *Police Practice and Research, 15*, 404–418. https://doi.org/10.1080/15614263.2013.829321

Visher, C. A., Harrell, A., Newmark, L., & Yahner, J. (2008). Reducing intimate partner violence: An evaluation of a comprehensive justice system-community collaboration. *Criminology & Public Policy, 7*, 495–523. https://doi.org/10.1111/j.1745-9133.2008.00524.x

Visher, C. A., Newmark, L. C., & Harrell, A. (2008). The evaluation of the judicial oversight demonstration: Findings and lessons on implementation. US Department of Justice, Office of Justice Programs, National Institute of Justice. https://www.nij.gov/publications/pages/publication-detail.aspx?ncjnumber=219077

Welsh, W. (2002). Evaluation of prison-based drug treatment in Pennsylvania: A research collaboration between the Pennsylvania Department of Corrections and the Center for Public Policy at Temple University: Final report. Philadelphia, PA: Center for Public Policy, Temple University. http://www.ncjrs.gov/App/publications/abstract.aspx?ID=197058

2

The University of Virginia's Institute of Law, Psychiatry, and Public Policy

RICHARD J. BONNIE, DANIEL C. MURRIE, AND HEATHER ZELLE ■

ORIGINS

The half-century of collaboration between the University of Virginia (UVA) and the Commonwealth of Virginia in mental health law took root in the early 1970s, just as mental health law was emerging as a distinct field of legal and scientific study encompassing both civil and criminal domains. Three fountainhead judicial decisions in 1972 made that year a convenient marker for the origins of the field and the creation of the Institute of Law, Psychiatry, and Public Policy (ILPPP): *Jackson v. Indiana* (the US Supreme Court's decision barring indeterminate commitment of criminal defendants found incompetent to stand trial), *Lessard v. Schmidt* (a West Virginia Supreme Court decision tightening the criteria for involuntary civil commitment), and *Wyatt v. Stickney* (a federal district court class action in Alabama in which Judge Frank Johnson proclaimed the legal rights of institutionalized psychiatric patients and established a structure for implementing them).

The first decade of collaboration between the University and the Commonwealth encompassed all of the challenges these landmark decisions raised, beginning with a contract to design a strategy for "deinstitutionalizing" pretrial forensic assessments and expanding by the end of the decade to include four aims: (1) training community mental health professionals to conduct pretrial forensic mental health evaluations, (2) advising the Department of Mental Health and Mental Retardation (now the Department of Behavioral Health and Developmental Services [DBHDS]) on legal reform of the civil commitment system, (3) implementing a program for protecting the rights of institutionalized psychiatric patients, and (4) developing a multimodal program of specialized professional education in mental health law.

LEADERSHIP AND INSPIRATION

From the start, this collaboration has been driven by a shared commitment to innovation. P. Browning Hoffman, MD, a psychiatrist, came to Charlottesville in 1971 with a joint appointment in the Schools of Medicine and Law after a fellowship at Yale under the tutelage of psychiatrist Jay Katz, a giant in the emerging fields of bioethics and health law. Dr. Hoffman began immediately to develop relationships with faculty in law and medicine with interests in health law and ethics, and he started an outpatient teaching clinic for forensic assessment, bringing faculty, residents, medical students, and law students into the same setting to discuss forensic evaluations. While getting acquainted with leaders in psychiatry in Virginia, Dr. Hoffman and the Commissioner of Mental Health and Mental Retardation, William Allerton, recognized the rich opportunities for collaboration arising out of deinstitutionalization as well as emerging legal regulation of psychiatric care in both public and private settings. An immediate priority in Virginia (as in many other states) was to develop a roadmap for shifting forensic assessments from the state hospitals to community mental health professionals. The implementation and eventual evolution of this plan is described in further depth here.

As the seeds for a university–state collaboration were planted in 1971–1973, the University's own vision of cross-professional collaboration in mental health, as well as its capacity to carry out innovations, grew markedly in the fall of 1973 when Richard J. Bonnie rejoined the Law School faculty after completing his service as Associate Director of the National Commission on Marijuana and Drug Abuse. Professors Hoffman and Bonnie jointly taught multiple courses in mental health law, including seminars built around the Forensic Clinic. (The primary seminar featured criminal cases, but a companion seminar was occasionally offered on civil cases.) They also created the ILPPP and initiated a post-JD fellowship in mental health law as well as a postresidency fellowship in forensic psychiatry. The first contract between the Department of Mental Health and Mental Retardation (now DBHDS) and the University was executed in 1975. Meanwhile, Dr. Hoffman and Professor Bonnie became involved in the American Psychiatric Association's policy development activities and in drafting amicus briefs for the US Supreme Court in a steady stream of cases involving forensic psychiatry and mental health law.

Unfortunately, this exciting time in the growth of the ILPPP and its innovative relationship with DBHDS was tragically interrupted in 1979, when Dr. Hoffman suddenly died at the age of 42. It is a testament to the strength and value of the activities initiated under Dr. Hoffman's leadership that the services provided by the ILPPP and its relationship with the Commonwealth did not miss a beat.

Fortunately, the University was able to recruit an emerging leader in law and psychology, John Monahan, to join the Law School faculty in 1980 and maintain collateral appointments in psychology and psychiatry.

CURRENT COLLABORATION

Leadership and Internal Structure

Although Richard Bonnie, whose primary appointment is in the UVA School of Law, served as ILPPP director since Dr. Hoffman's death in 1979, many other aspects of the ILPPP structure and leadership have changed over the years. The current ILPPP structure has evolved to include two branches. The first focuses primarily on forensic mental health issues in the criminal justice system, including a forensic clinic and the long-standing state contract to train Virginia clinicians in forensic evaluation. This section has been led since 2008 by a forensic/clinical psychologist: Daniel Murrie, PhD, a professor in the Medical School's Department of Psychiatry and Neurobehavioral Sciences. The second branch of the ILPPP focuses primarily on broader mental health law and policy. This branch has been led since 2015 by a psychologist/attorney: Heather Zelle, JD, PhD, an assistant professor of research in the Department of Public Health Sciences. The organizational chart does not tell the whole story, of course. As is often the case in academic settings, senior faculty play important collegial and supervisory roles in the ILPPP as they carry out their teaching and research obligations in their respective schools. John Monahan (Law School) and Janet Warren (Department of Psychiatry and Neurobehavioral Sciences) have contributed immeasurably to the accomplishments of the ILPPP. Historically, excellent forensic psychiatrists (i.e., Park Dietz, Steven K. Hoge, and Eileen Ryan) also served as medical directors of the ILPPP.

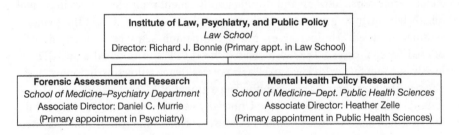

Contractual Arrangements

Just as the ILPPP has developed two branches with distinct foci, the ILPPP–DBHDS collaboration has also evolved to include two separate contracts covering two separate domains of work, each involving somewhat different relations to

DBHDS. For example, the ILPPP contract that supports forensic consultation and forensic training for clinicians is overseen by the state forensic director. Currently, the ILPPP contract that addresses mental health policy research is overseen by the deputy commissioner of compliance, regulatory, and legislative affairs and involves coordination with other department leadership (i.e., deputy or assistant commissioners, division directors, etc.) as needed for contracted projects. Of course, each contract requires different coordination and relationships with other stakeholders. For example, the mental health policy research team has an ongoing collaboration with the DBHDS's data scientists and analysts and has worked with the community behavioral health services department for a project addressing psychiatric advance directives. In addition, the mental health policy research team has collaborated—individually and collectively—with local outpatient mental health providers around the state as well as stakeholder agencies such as hospital associations and mental health advocacy groups.

Like most state contracts, ILPPP–DBHDS funding has ebbed and flowed corresponding to the health of the state budget. But it has generally decreased, particularly in light of inflation. In the early years, the forensic services contract supported multiple faculty positions to aid in training, but, for the past few decades, the contract has covered only basic training costs and small fractions of faculty time. By contrast, the sources of funding for the mental health policy branch of the ILPPP have varied substantially over the years, depending on the nature, stability, and size of research grants. For many years, for example, the ILPPP was a key research site for studies conducted by the MacArthur Research Networks on Mental Health Law (1988–1998) and Mandated Community Treatment (2001–2010), both directed by John Monahan. Since the MacArthur funding ended, however, the work of the mental health policy research branch has largely been supported by the DBHDS mental health law reform contract. As noted in the "Significant Changes in the Collaboration" section later in this chapter, however, the ILPPP is currently exploring ways to provide some stability to its staffing and further diversify its funding sources.

As other chapters throughout this book have emphasized, state funding often remains stagnant, and a challenge to most state contracts is the need to consistently do more work with less funding. Another important factor in the negotiation of funding with the state can be leadership turnover and, as agency priorities change, uneven commitment to the value of the partnership. A key challenge is maintaining the agency leadership's understanding of the unique subject matter expertise and institutional memory provided by the ILPPP, as well as its ready access to the University's expertise in adjacent disciplines. A related issue is that newly arriving state agency leaders often assume, incorrectly, that the ILPPP's research activity is independently funded by the University and that ILPPP expertise would remain available despite budget-driven gaps in DBHDS funding. The DBHDS contracts with the ILPPP on an annual basis, so these conversations can be a yearly exercise in attempting to maintain a workable budget and scope of work.

DOMAINS OF COLLABORATION

Collaboration between state government and universities has advantages in several broad domains: policy innovation, program implementation and oversight, professional training, and public education. These advantages are magnified when the university contribution is interdisciplinary; in the ILPPP's case, this involves primarily expertise from the law school as well as the medical school, but also some collaboration with faculty from other university departments and with the bar, the judiciary, and professional societies. This section describes ILPPP activities in three domains: (1) policy development, (2) forensic training and related activities, and (3) public and professional education in mental health law.

Policy Development

Designing solutions to specific policy problems is a particularly promising basis for university–state government collaboration. As noted earlier, the ILPPP–DBHDS relationship was first created to design, implement, and evaluate the potential for community-based forensic services, thereby facilitating a transition from a hospital-based system for evaluating criminal defendants to a community-based system. Key challenges included creating a curriculum, developing a plan for assessing trainee knowledge and skills, designing a new legal structure to govern the system, and securing its enactment by the General Assembly. These activities, initiated in 1975 and completed around 1980, still provide the basic legal infrastructure for training community evaluators in forensic assessment and for oversight of the program jointly by the ILPPP and the DBHDS Office of Forensic Services. In turn, this widely respected program also provides a stable foundation for the multifaceted collaboration between the ILPPP and the DBHDS.

An example of policy innovation in the 1980s and 1990s was the development of the DBHDS "human rights program" to protect the rights of institutionalized persons and—as the locus of services moved to the community—to protect the rights of clients receiving services in the community. Building on Judge Johnson's decision in *Wyatt* and the brief federal Mental Health Systems initiative carried out during the Carter Administration, many states, including Virginia, launched mental health "patient advocacy" programs. As explained in greater depth later, structural independence from the services system and adequate funding for investigation and complaint resolution are essential elements of successful advocacy programs, and the ILPPP played a key role in designing the legal architecture of an advocacy program internally at DBHDS to complement an external program with litigation authority (Virginia Office for Protection and Advocacy, now the disAbility Law Center of Virginia [dLCV]).

ILPPP policy innovation in the twenty-first century has focused on improving and reforming crisis services and facilitating treatment engagement among persons with chronic mental illness living in the community—the "unfinished business" of deinstitutionalization. One key initiative was laying the legal foundation for use of mental health advance directives and launching the only effort to implement advance directives in routine community care. This uphill battle continues. Another key twenty-first century initiative has been developing the legal foundation for and implementing mandatory outpatient treatment—also a project that remains in its earliest stages. Each of these initiatives was grounded in the path-breaking work of the MacArthur Foundation Research Network on Mandated Community Treatment, led by John Monahan.

Not surprisingly, a major focus of the ILPPP–DBHDS relationship between 2005 and 2020 has been designing and implementing a comprehensive array of crisis services and the accompanying legal requirements for assessment, transportation, decision-making, intensive treatment, and community support. These challenges face virtually every state. In this context, the ILPPP–DBHDS partnership is borrowing innovations developed and implemented elsewhere rather than inventing its own. What is most noteworthy regarding this sequence of collaborative activities is that they have drawn the ILPPP and the DBHDS into health services research and implementation sciences—outside the ILPPP's traditional domain of legal design.

Forensic Training

After a new policy or program is created, implementation, oversight, and quality assurance are typically absorbed by the public services system or contracted out to private entities. An academic institution does not typically add value in these situations if the skills are fungible with those of other service providers. However, tasks that require interdisciplinary expertise and professional neutrality (i.e., being "above the fray") may be exceptions to this proposition. One example is providing advice and quality assurance in forensic assessments (to providers as well as the courts).

An early and primary focus of the ILPPP was a program designed to provide training in forensic evaluation to psychologists and psychiatrists. Such training was crucial to the mission of "deinstitutionalizing" forensic services—moving most forensic evaluations outside of the state psychiatric hospitals and into jails or community clinics. The pilot project for community-based forensic services was established by the Virginia General Assembly with a House Joint Resolution passed in 1980. Simultaneous, statewide implementation was not feasible, so the ILPPP developed a pilot project involving several jurisdictions, which allowed for a quasi-experimental design (comparing the pilot jurisdictions with those that operated with services as usual). The pilot project—detailed thoroughly in *Community Mental Health Centers and the Courts: An Evaluation of Community-Based Forensic Services* (Melton, Weithorn, & Slobogin, 1985)—was a clear success.

In short, the pilot project revealed that community clinicians could be trained to a high level of forensic expertise and that community-based services could reduce costly hospital admissions for forensic evaluations. Indeed, the project revealed "strong support for the notion that a community-based system of forensic services results in substantial fiscal savings while reducing unnecessary intrusions into the defendant's interests in bail and a speedy trial" (Melton et al., 1985, p. 43). Further, the pilot project that studied this effort documented numerous positive outcomes in terms of the work products (forensic evaluation reports) produced, state funds saved, and even expertise developed among state clinicians (whom testing showed were performing similarly to a national sample of board-certified forensic experts; Melton et al., 1985). The curriculum, or clinician training materials, developed for this pilot project eventually evolved into the leading textbook for forensic evaluations, now in its fourth edition (Melton et al., 2018).

Ultimately, Virginia expanded the pilot project throughout the state and made related changes to statute and policy. For example, the statutes governing competence, sanity, and certain other questions related to forensic mental health (e.g., sentencing of capital offenders and sexual offenders) were all revised to indicate that any evaluator appointed to perform the evaluation must have appropriate training. Such specialized training has since been available through the ILPPP (at very low cost to DBHDS staff, but also open to others) annually and includes:

- Basic Forensic Evaluation, addressing competence, sanity, expert testimony, and related issues (5 days)
- Violence Risk Assessment (1 day)
- Evaluating those charged with sexual offenses (2 days)
- Evaluations at capital sentencing (2 days)
- Evaluating (for risk management) those acquitted as Not Guilty by Reason of Insanity (1 day).

Over the years, the state developed a similar training curriculum for the forensic evaluation of juveniles that includes:

- Basic Forensic Evaluation of Juveniles (5 days)
- Violence Risk Assessment with Juveniles (1 day).

Each of these routine training sessions is directed by ILPPP faculty, but each training features many different speakers, including ILPPP faculty and other regional or national experts.

Beyond the standard curriculum or sequences of courses just listed, the ILPPP collaborates with the DBHDS to provide approximately five additional "special topic" training sessions (usually with national experts) addressing any further, or advanced, training needs in a given year. Thus, the ILPPP–DBHDS collaboration typically provides at least 20 days of training to forensic mental health professionals each year. Most of the routine training sessions (i.e., those offered annually) serve classes of approximately 30 clinicians each, though class sizes for very specialized forensic services (e.g., capital sentencing evaluations) are usually smaller, and class sizes for additional "special topic" training sessions that are not offered annually are much larger.

THE DBHDS FORENSIC OVERSIGHT PROGRAM

Closely related to the longstanding goal of providing forensic training for Virginia clinicians, a complementary objective recently emerged for the ILPPP-DBHDS partnership: an oversight system to improve the quality of court-ordered forensic evaluations. The statewide oversight program—unique to Virginia as far as we know—is based in the central office of the DBHDS forensic division (not the ILPPP) and employs one Oversight Director as well as support staff. Upon creation of the oversight system, DBHDS prompted modifications to the Virginia statutes guiding competence and sanity evaluations. For example, Virginia Code Section § 19.2-169.5 now states, " . . . in all cases, the evaluator shall send a redacted copy of the report removing references to the defendant's name, date of birth, case number, and court of jurisdiction to the Commissioner of Behavioral Health and Developmental Services for the purpose of peer review to establish and maintain the list of approved evaluators . . . " Therefore, to be in compliance with the Code of Virginia, all evaluators who submit a court-ordered competence or sanity report of an adult defendant must also submit a redacted copy to the Virginia DBHDS.

Though the oversight system operates almost entirely within DBHDS, the ILPPP helps in several training tasks (e.g., ILPPP faculty serve on the panels reviewing reports, and then help translate findings from the oversight system into training goals and content for the ILPPP forensic trainings). Moreover, the ILPPP collaborates with DBHDS in research tasks made possible through the oversight system. The unique program that collects reports from court-ordered evaluations on a state-wide basis has allowed for some of the largest existing studies of forensic evaluation report quality and practices (e.g., Gardner et al., 2018; Murrie et al., 2020) as well as studies addressing broader criminal justice issues that intersect with forensic evaluations (e.g., Gardner et al., in press; Murrie et al., in press). These inform Virginia training and practice, but may have broader significance as well.

THE ILPPP FORENSIC CLINIC

Closely intertwined with the clinical training mission of the ILPPP was the development of a forensic psychiatry clinic. In the 1970s, the ILPPP established a small forensic clinic for the sole purpose of conducting forensic evaluations that could be used for teaching purposes. Clinical faculty (psychologists and psychiatrists) led the evaluations, often with law students observing. The interdisciplinary faculty discussed cases at case conferences or similar clinic meetings, and the grainy video recordings of the interviews became aids for the contracted annual training sessions.

Not until the 1990s did it become clear that the clinic could expand beyond a narrow role of generating a few teaching examples and also serve Virginia by providing court-ordered or even privately retained evaluations on a more frequent basis. Psychologist Gary Hawk oversaw the clinic and the training program and increasingly accepted forensic evaluations, which eventually began to serve as a source of revenue to support faculty. Because the clinic had the benefit of a multidisciplinary team (with access to a forensic psychologist, psychiatrist, social worker, and attorneys) it became somewhat of a niche practice addressing more complex, challenging, or high-profile cases.

In recent years, the clinic has expanded substantially. From 2008 to 2020, the clinic, directed by psychologist Daniel Murrie, expanded from a few dozen evaluations each year to several hundred each year, and revenue increased by roughly 10-fold. This allowed (and required) staffing to expand from one faculty psychologist and one postdoctoral fellow to several faculty and fellows. Thus, full-time clinic faculty (originally just one psychologist and one postdoctoral fellow) now include three psychologists (all former ILPPP postdoctoral fellows), a neuropsychologist, and multiple postdoctoral fellows. This expansion allowed for greater specialization among the faculty—each develops one or more specialized forensic practice niches—which enhances clinical services and also provides further specialized expertise for ILPPP training sessions. The increasing case volume and substantial growth of the clinic has provided substantial increase in revenue during an era when state funding has decreased (described elsewhere in this chapter), allowing for added positions for trainees (i.e., additional postdoctoral fellowships in forensic psychology) and expanding the training mission of the ILPPP.

Fellowships and Other Specialized Training

Although the ILPPP clinic had always welcomed students and trainees (from law, psychiatry, psychology, and related disciplines) to observe cases or assist with evaluations under supervision, it was not until recent decades that the clinic developed formal fellowships. The fellowships were not sponsored by the state training contract (in contrast to University of Massachusetts Medical School, described in Chapter 3, for example). However, the UVA medical school oversees certain training fellowships—including some in collaboration with Western State Hospital—and ultimately designated certain fellowships for forensic psychology and forensic psychiatry. Thus, most fellows receive diverse forensic training that spans a state psychiatric hospital and the private, university-based clinic at ILPPP (though some fellows are based only in ILPPP). Although not funded by DBHDS, the fellowships inevitably benefit DBHDS and the Commonwealth of Virginia. For example, they attract some of the strongest candidates from across the country, who then work for part of their fellowship year in DBHDS facilities and then (in some cases) take positions in the Virginia system (including DBHDS facilities) upon graduation.

Public and Professional Education in Mental Health Law

A third area of ongoing collaboration between DBHDS and ILPPP is professional and public education on legal aspects of mental health law. Mental health law was a newly developing field in the 1970s and 1980s, and everyone involved (professors in the law school as well as attorneys in Office of the Attorney General (OAG) responsible for advising DBHDS) was on a fairly steep learning curve—the demand for advice intensified at all levels of government and among public and private clinicians, lawyers, and judges. Beginning in 1981, the ILPPP–DBHDS contract included support for the ILPPP's "newsletter" on *Developments in Mental Health Law*, designed to summarize case law and legislative activity (in Virginia and elsewhere) for administrators, interested clinicians, judges, and interested members of the bar. In addition, the ILPPP–DBHDS contract funded an annual conference or symposium on topics of current interest. Both of these activities continue four decades later.

SIGNIFICANT CHANGES IN THE COLLABORATION

As noted earlier, areas of collaboration between the ILPPP and the DBHDS include policy development and program implementation. For both domains, the ILPPP has provided research services grounded in legal knowledge as well as clinical and legal advice. Although the ILPPP continues to provide those services, the method has evolved in recent years. For a time, the extent of ILPPP's collaboration on these fronts waxed and waned with the changing intensity of executive and/ or legislative attention to mental health in Virginia. In recent years, however, a period of concentrated attention by the Virginia General Assembly has prompted greater attention by both state branches to the role of data in policymaking. As a result, the ILPPP has been actively engaged with both the executive and legislative branches. The attention also spurred the DBHDS to grow its capacity for harnessing and applying data to its decision-making and oversight of services.

Interestingly, the simultaneous developments led to a need for change in the collaboration between the ILPPP and the DBHDS, including substantive changes to the mental health policy research contract. The DBHDS expanded its ability to undertake some of the general surveillance data analysis that the ILPPP had provided for several years and to conduct analyses with its growing warehouse of data. The ILPPP hoped to sustain a long-term role in policy research to complement a rather cyclic attention to mental health policy and implementation.

The contractual agreement between the ILPPP and the DBHDS thus needed to be reimagined at this crossroads: it could no longer consist of essentially the same basic "products" each year in the form of annual surveillance reports and the like. Recognizing the DBHDS's capacity to conduct such work on its own and the redundancy of contracting with the ILPPP to provide largely similar work, a new scope of work was needed, one that was more responsive to current foci of the DBHDS and made the most of the ILPPP's expertise. In addition to renegotiating the contract with the DBHDS, the ILPPP also sought to shore up its workforce stability and infrastructure by partnering with another department in the University's medical school—the Department of Public Health Sciences. The expertise of public health faculty and staff aligns with the data-based, public health approach to mental health law that the ILPPP applies in its work with the DBHDS. Furthermore, integrating public health faculty and staff provides stability for the ILPPP, which has at times seen its Mental Health Policy Research team size fluctuate starkly based on contractual funding. The ultimate goal of this budding model is to sustain the ILPPP as a robust policy research collaborator for the DBHDS (and perhaps other stakeholders to come)—a collaborator that is responsive to the DBHDS's needs, is able to take on research of innovations in mental health policy, and sustains a base level of research capacity to assess the effects of policy changes. Additionally, the continuing collaboration allows the ILPPP to manage projects that require the "professional neutrality" mentioned earlier in this chapter, as many of the policies and programs currently under development in Virginia entail active involvement by the legislative branch and other stakeholders beyond the DBHDS. Internally at the University, the ILPPP's partnership with Public Health Sciences has the added benefit of training masters-level public health professionals with knowledge in mental health policy and research.

STRUCTURAL INNOVATIONS AND CHALLENGES

The ILPPP's affiliation with a law school and its intensive engagement in policy development raises occasional tension between the academic and professional independence of its faculty and its obligations to its long-term contractual partner, DBHDS. The somewhat unusual ILPPP experience also highlights the pervasive engagement of all three branches of government in mental health law policy-making as well as its daily administration. For illustrative purposes, we describe two topics: (a) ILPPP's relationship with the OAG and (b) its role as a resource for the General Assembly, the Supreme Court of Virginia, and the Executive Branch—a highly useful role that can nonetheless be a source of tension and conflict.

ILPPP and the Office of the Attorney General

The ILPPP's relationship with the OAG has evolved over time. It is important to re-emphasize that the ILPPP–DBHDS partnership took root just as the field of mental health law, including laws governing forensic services, was taking shape. As the Attorney General's Office and the Institute faculty were educating themselves about the evolving body of mental health law, they were engaging in ongoing collegial interchange and public discussion about the meaning of new cases or statutes. However, it was critical for everyone to understand that only the OAG had the authority to give legal advice to state agencies and employees. For these reasons, the OAG was a party to the ILPPP–DBHDS contract in the early phase of the ILPPP–DBHDS relationship and was given the opportunity to review all law-related training materials directed to state employees.

After this formative period, as the law became more detailed and complex and the number of attorneys in the OAG specializing in mental health law increased, uncertainties regarding the respective roles of the OAG and the ILPPP attorneys evaporated. The OAG attorneys are the acknowledged authorities on interpretation of state law, while the ILPPP attorneys focus on exploring ambiguities in existing law and identifying opportunities and needs for legal reform.

The situation was more complicated for local officials. A key element of services system change during the 1980s was the development of 40 local community mental health services agencies (called Community Service Boards in Virginia). Because the community agencies are part of local governments, the OAG is not responsible for providing direct legal advice to those boards, who are served by city and county attorneys. In this respect, part of the Institute's role has been to collaborate with both the OAG and local government attorneys as the system has become more sophisticated and the fraternity of specialists has grown.

Facilitation of Mental Health Law Reform

One of the ILPPP's most interesting—and challenging—roles has been to serve as a catalyst or facilitator for mental health law reform and sometimes as a bridge between executive, legislative, and judicial bodies. Indeed, this may have been one of the ILPPP's greatest accomplishments, albeit one fraught with structural risks and ambiguities. Given its 40-year history, this subject would fill a book by itself, but a few illustrations will suffice for purposes of this chapter.

EXECUTIVE BRANCH INITIATIVES

As mentioned earlier, one of the first developments in mental health reform in the 1970s was the creation of advocacy systems for protecting the rights of institutionalized psychiatric patients in the wake of *Wyatt v. Stickney* in 1972. Virginia, like many other states, opted for an "internal" advocacy system for monitoring and enforcing patient rights. Each facility director was responsible for hiring a patient advocate and for appointing local citizen members of a local human rights committee (LHRC). In addition, the Commissioner was responsible for appointing citizen members of a state human rights committee (SHRC) to provide statewide oversight. When the system was established, Dr. Browning Hoffman was appointed by Commissioner Leo E. Kirven Jr. to the SHRC. After Dr. Hoffman's untimely death in 1979, Professor Bonnie was appointed to take his seat and became SHRC chair in 1980.

After the enabling legislation was enacted in 1977, the State Board of Mental Health and Mental Retardation (now the State Board of Behavioral Health and Developmental Services) adopted fairly bare-bones regulations to implement the statute. Although Dr. Hoffman and Professor Bonnie supported the basic design of an internal system—with full access to all patients and all facility employees—it became clear to them that the original Virginia structure lacked sufficient independence: the facility advocates were appointed by the facility director, as were the members of the LHRCs.

After several years of experience, the SHRC established a subcommittee to develop improved regulations with more detailed substantive protections and a new structure providing greater independence for the advocates and for the

local committees. Under the revised regulations, the facility advocates were appointed by the DBHDS central office and the LHRC members were appointed
by the SHRC. Members of the SHRC were, in turn, appointed by the State Board
(whose members were appointed by the Governor). ILPPP staff provided direct
support to the SHRC and, in turn, to the State Board in the development of these
regulations. Since Professor Bonnie's tenure on the SHRC ended, the ILPPP has
not had a formal role in the administration of the DBHDS human rights program.
From a historical standpoint, it is also important to note that the Commonwealth
also has a robust independent advocacy organization, the dLCV.

ASSISTANCE TO THE LEGISLATURE

Ideas for legislation often originate in executive agencies and eventually become
part of the Governor's legislative program or are embraced by legislators themselves without formal gubernatorial endorsement. Over the decades, many legislative innovations in mental health law have emerged from task forces or work
groups established in DBHDS with leadership or participation by ILPPP, especially in the forensic services domain. Examples included the implementation of
community-based forensic evaluations, commitment and conditional release of
insanity acquittees, and several revisions of the statutory procedures for emergency mental health evaluations.

Given the expertise in mental health law at the ILPPP, members of the legislature
often seek advice and consultation. Often this has been informal collaboration in
developing bills. However, some initiatives have been much more structured and
have involved DBHDS (and the ILPPP–DBHDS contract) in a formal way. Several
examples involving civil commitment reform illustrate the creative variations that
have been deployed over the years.

In 1982, the General Assembly established a special "joint subcommittee"
chaired by a young member of the House of Delegates with a particular interest
in civil commitment reform. Eventually a partnership developed between that
legislator and Professor Bonnie, who was then chairing the SHRC. In addition,
empirical research (observations of commitment hearings) was provided with
support from the Virginia Bar Foundation. Although the civil commitment overhaul proposed by the joint subcommittee was not enacted (due to the projected
cost), the partnership eventually produced a long overdue reform of the statutes
governing psychiatric hospitalization of minors in 1990.

Historically, the most ambitious (and most interesting) collaboration between
the ILPPP and DBHDS involved an overhaul of the civil commitment process in the wake of the tragic mass shooting at Virginia Tech in April 2007 (see
Bonnie, Reinhard, Hamilton, & McGarvey, 2009; http://www.courts.state.va.us/
programs/concluded/cmh/home.html). This collaboration had been initiated by
the Chief Justice of the Supreme Court of Virginia in December of 2005, when he
asked Professor Bonnie to chair a Commission on Mental Health Law Reform.
Ultimately, the Commission and its five task forces were drawn from all three
branches of government and key stakeholder organizations. Funding for the
Commission's research was provided through a contract between DBHDS and

ILPPP. The Commission held its first meeting in October 2006, expecting a 2-year study of the process. However, the pace was accelerated after the Virginia Tech tragedy, and the General Assembly enacted major legal reforms during the 2008 and 2009 sessions and appropriated a $40 million "down payment" for services improvements (Bonnie et al., 2009).

Although a national recession interrupted progress, and the Commission expired in 2011, another major reform initiative was launched during the 2014 legislative session following the tragic death of "Gus" Deeds, the son of state Senator Creigh Deeds. The General Assembly established a new Joint Subcommittee to Study Mental Health Service in the Twenty-First Century chaired by Senator Deeds. Once again, DBHDS contracted with ILPPP to provide additional research support for the new legislative inquiry. These successive collaborations between the three branches of state government and the ILPPP were unorthodox and are not likely to be replicated. However, research collaboration on mental health law reform continues in a more traditional format under an ILPPP–DBHDS contract supporting agency priorities, such as improving the system's capacity to provide mandatory outpatient treatment.

One of the reforms developed at the ILPPP for the Supreme Court's Commission was a comprehensive overhaul of the Health Care Decisions Act that included detailed provisions governing advance directives relating to mental health care. The act included a number of important (and intriguing) legal innovations, including a "Ulysses clause" (a provision executed when an individual has capacity in anticipation of a time when that person will lack capacity, thereby enabling a person to authorize treatment over later objection while decisionally incapable). Enactment of this important law was only the beginning of a continuing effort to educate the public, mental health consumers and their families, and mental health clinicians and other service providers about the law, as well as to develop models for assisting consumers to execute such advance directives. This is one of the areas where ILPPP and DBHDS have collaborated on implementation, a still-unfolding process (Kemp, Zelle, & Bonnie, 2015; Zelle, Kemp, & Bonnie, 2015).

CLOSING THOUGHTS

Partnerships between universities and state governments offer significant advantages to both parties. For the university, such a partnership can provide hands-on learning experiences for students, trainees, and fellows in delivering services or, depending on the type of program, in translating policy ideas into practice. Under the best of circumstances, such a partnership can also provide the university with a stable source of support for the academic mission. For the state government, an academic partnership can be useful in training service providers and managers and can assure ready access to the expertise needed to address policy problems as they arise. At its best, an academic partnership also provides opportunities for research and consultation on service delivery, program implementation, and policy development.

Although we are by no means objective observers, we believe that both UVA and the Commonwealth of Virginia have benefited from a long-term partnership first forged in the early stage of the "revolution" in mental health law that emerged during the late 1960s and early 1970s. This partnership has spawned genuine innovation in forensic services and mental health policy development and has provided a laboratory for research by generations of students from a variety of academic disciplines. The ILPPP–DBHDS collaboration on forensic services has been a highly successful investment in Virginia and has served as a model for other states. That said, however, the Virginia partnership has experienced obstacles and challenges along the way, the most worrisome being an underinvestment in research and uneven state funding attributable to the vicissitudes of the economy and the changing priorities of agency leaders.

Virginia's partnership between DBHDS and the ILPPP has also encountered unique structural challenges relating to its connections, both formal and informal, with all three branches of state government. Interbranch collaboration of this kind is not likely to occur—or to continue—without a spirit of mutual trust between the state agency and the university. It seems unlikely that a university-agency partnership of this kind can sustain its policy influence in the absence of a shared perception that the University's expertise and independence offer something of value. UVA's experience may be unique in this respect because the ILPPP and DBHDS have been responding—as partners—to ongoing changes in the services system and the law over many decades as the field itself was developing and as new challenges arose. In retrospect, the ILPPP's stable leadership may have provided continuity for mental health law reform during a period of rapid change together with ongoing transitions in the state's leadership. Whether this relationship continues, and, if so, how it adapts to changing political circumstances, remain to be seen.

REFERENCES

Bonnie, R. J., Reinhard, J. S., Hamilton, P., & McGarvey, E. L. (2009). Mental health system transformation after the Virginia Tech tragedy. *Health Affairs, 28*(3), 793–804. doi:10.1377/hlthaff.28.3.793

Jackson v. Indiana, 406 US 715 (1972).

Gardner, B. O., Murrie, D. C., & Torres, A. N. (in press). The impact of misdemeanor arrests in forensic mental health services: A state-wide review of Virginia sanity evaluations. *Law and Human Behavior.*

Gardner, B. O., Murrie, D. C., & Torres, A. (2018). Insanity findings and evaluation practices: A state-wide review of court-ordered reports. *Behavioral Sciences & the Law, 36,* 303–316.

Kemp, K., Zelle, H., & Bonnie, R. J. (2015). Embedding advance directives in routine care for persons with serious mental illness: The challenge of implementation. *Psychiatric Services, 66,* 10–14. doi:10.1176/appi.ps.201400276

Lessard v. Schmidt, 349 F. Supp. 1078 (E.D. Wis. 1972).

Melton, G. B., Petrila, J., Poythress, N. G., Slobogin, C., Otto, R. K., Mossman D., & Condie, L. O. (2018). *Psychological evaluations for the courts: A handbook for mental health professionals and lawyers* (4th ed.). New York: Guilford.

Melton, G. B., Weithorn, L. A., & Slobogin, C. (1985). *Community mental health centers and the courts: An evaluation of community-based forensic services.* Lincoln: University of Nebraska Press.

Murrie, D. C., Gardner, B. O., & Torres, A. N. (in press). The impact of misdemeanor arrests in forensic mental health services: A state-wide review of Virginia Competence to Stand Trial evaluations. *Psychology, Public Policy, and Law.*

Murrie, D. C., Gardner, B. O., & Torres, A. N. (2020). Competency to stand trial evaluations: A state-wide review of court-ordered reports. *Behavioral Sciences and the Law*, 1–19.

Wyatt v. Stickney, 325 F.Supp. 781 (M.D. Ala. 1971).

Zelle, H., Kemp, K., & Bonnie, R. J. (2015). Advance directives for mental health care: Innovation in law, policy, and practice. *Psychiatric Services, 66*, 7–9. doi:10.1176/appi.ps.201400435

3

The Designated Forensic Professional Program in Massachusetts

IRA K. PACKER AND THOMAS GRISSO ■

Collaboration between universities and public behavioral health systems has been important in the Commonwealth of Massachusetts. This chapter describes the particular collaboration between the University of Massachusetts Medical School (UMMS) and the Massachusetts Department of Mental Health (DMH).

PURPOSE AND INITIATION OF COLLABORATION

In 1985, the Commonwealth of Massachusetts faced a dilemma. There was an increasing number of defendants with mental illness being arraigned and in need of evaluations for competence to stand trial (CST) and/or criminal responsibility (CR). There was only a small cadre of psychiatrists who were available at the courthouses to conduct these evaluations. Furthermore, most of the psychiatrists were not specifically trained to conduct such forensic evaluations. In addition, once the defendant was sent to a state hospital for a more in-depth evaluation, most of those attending psychiatrists were not trained in forensic psychiatry, so the quality of reports being sent back to the courts was poor. In response to this growing problem, the Massachusetts legislature convened a committee to make recommendations. The result was the development of a Division of Forensic Mental Health within DMH, headed by an Assistant Commissioner, with a mandate to develop a high-quality system to provide forensic evaluations to the courts (Fein et al., 1991).

At the same time, the Legislature modified existing statutes to allow psychologists qualified by the DMH to conduct court-ordered evaluations of CST and CR. Until 1985, only psychiatrists, or psychologists working at the maximum-security Bridgewater State Hospital, were authorized to conduct such evaluations, but this new mandate required development of a much-expanded workforce. This new legislation greatly increased the potential number of psychologists available to conduct these forensic evaluations at courthouses and at DMH hospitals. Although these important legislative enactments opened the door to systemic change, the challenge was ensuring that psychologists hired for this function were appropriately qualified and trained.

To address this challenge, the newly appointed Assistant Commissioner for Forensic Services (Robert Fein, PhD, an American Board of Forensic Psychology [ABFP] board-certified forensic psychologist who had served as co-medical director at Bridgewater State Hospital) turned to the Psychiatry Department of the state's public sector medical school: tUMMS. UMMS had recently developed a Law and Psychiatry Program, headed by a prominent psychiatrist and researcher (Paul Appelbaum, MD). The expectation was that the Law and Psychiatry Program, with its excellent national reputation, would attract qualified professionals to develop and maintain a statewide training program in forensic mental health. Within one year, UMMS was able to attract a nationally recognized forensic psychologist and researcher (Thomas Grisso, PhD) to join the Law and Psychiatry Program. Beginning in 1987, he worked with DMH to develop a training program for public-sector forensic professionals, develop and implement standards for forensic reports, and certify individual practitioners as competent to conduct these evaluations.

This collaboration between DMH and UMMS resulted in two major training efforts. First, it resulted in the development of the Designated Forensic Professional (DFP) Program, with the following purposes: (1) disseminating standards for forensic evaluations (with a focus on CST and CR), (2) providing didactic forensic training for practitioners who would perform court-ordered evaluations in the Commonwealth's courts and forensic inpatient units, (3) overseeing a mentoring process for candidates for certification, (4) developing a written examination that all candidates must pass, (5) developing a process whereby candidates would submit written work samples to a committee for approval before they could practice independently as DFPs, and (6) providing ongoing training and education to forensic practitioners. Although initially focused only on psychologists, the program was ultimately expanded to include training and certification of forensic psychiatrists in the public sector system as well (104 CMR 33.03, 2019).

Second, it provided UMMS with resources to develop a postdoctoral training program in forensic psychology, attracting students nationwide to receive one year of specialized forensic training and potentially (for some, at least) to obtain their first jobs in the Massachusetts courts and forensic hospitals. These resources included not only funding for faculty, but also funding for a postdoctoral fellow. Over the years the funding was increased to provide capacity for two postdoctoral fellows (now called Forensic Psychology Residents). In addition, the infrastructure allowed for additional trainees to be funded through contracts with other agencies and providers, so the program has grown to provide three slots annually.

This collaborative model proved to be attractive to psychologists who were interested in developing specialized expertise in forensic psychology. As there were limited opportunities at that time for psychologists to obtain this training in graduate schools or internships, the prospects for either on-the-job training or a postdoctoral fellowship at UMMS were attractive to potential applicants. Furthermore, unlike some other states that contracted directly with private practitioners to perform forensic evaluations, all forensic evaluators serving Massachusetts court clinics and hospitals were either state employees or employed by vendors who contracted with state agencies. Thus, the training and certification program was perceived as a benefit rather than a restriction on private practice. In addition, the certification was considered an achievement of status rather than an imposition. This was particularly true for young psychologists as yet without forensic specialization training.

This program was not as attractive to a small group of clinical psychologists working in state hospitals, who were less interested in becoming forensic evaluators. In the context of the changing landscape, several of them were required by the state to conduct forensic evaluations as part of their job duties. Unlike the majority of psychologists involved in the training, who enthusiastically entered the field, this group included individuals who were mandated to undergo forensic assessment training in order to keep their jobs. Within this group, several either did not complete the certification program or eventually left.

For psychiatrists, the certification process did not begin until several years after the psychology certification had been implemented. By then, the value of the certification status had been established. In addition, by that time, those psychiatrists applying for certification were employed by DMH or one of the vendors, and many had completed the Forensic Psychiatry Fellowship at UMMS.

NATURE OF THE COLLABORATION

The original DFP program was focused predominantly on providing forensic training to psychologists and psychiatrists working in District and Superior Courts (with adults), although eventually it also addressed juvenile courts. In 1999, a decision was made by DMH to develop a separate training program for juvenile court clinicians. This enhancement reflected the developmental issues impacting the assessment of adolescents, the different values and processes in juvenile court, and an expansion of the mandate to broaden the scope of training—to include master's level clinicians who could conduct some of the juvenile court evaluations that did not involve CST or CR. This expansion occurred in 1999, 12 years after the initiation of the DFP program. Again, DMH turned to UMMS to develop this training and certification. Dr. Grisso, who specialized in juvenile forensic work, agreed to take on this new task. UMMS then recruited Dr. Ira Packer, also an ABFP board-certified forensic psychologist and former Assistant Commissioner of Forensic Services in Massachusetts, to direct the DFP program. The process of forensic training for juvenile court clinicians was modeled closely after the original process for providing forensic training of DFPs.

This collaboration has continued for more than 30 years. The initial impetus was the need to attract psychologists and provide them with relevant specialized forensic training required by the Commonwealth. That goal has been met, as forensic psychologists now conduct the vast majority of public-sector forensic evaluations for CST and CR at courthouses and in the state hospitals. This success has allowed DMH to focus on maintaining quality control, updating standards, and expansion into other areas. Notably, the ability of UMMS as an academic institution to attract professionals with specialized expertise has provided a resource for DMH to obtain specialized training sessions and consultations in the area of violence risk assessment. UMMS faculty have been involved with the state agency in developing a policy addressing the risk assessment of involuntarily hospitalized individuals with significant violence histories. In addition, DMH has utilized UMMS faculty to provide training sessions on violence risk assessment and management to its community providers. This training was initially funded through a federal block grant, which was funneled from DMH to UMMS, but has continued with support from state funding.

The development of these training sessions for community providers followed a similar process to the initial development of the DFP program. The state agency identified a need: as the number of continuing care inpatient psychiatric hospital beds declined, many individuals with mental illness and histories of violence were discharged to community providers. These providers were tasked with serving individuals being discharged from state hospitals, but they did not have specialized experience in or knowledge of how to assess and manage the growing number who had more significant risk issues. DMH was able to turn to the Law and Psychiatry program to develop annual training sessions for community providers. DMH and community providers identified specific needs (e.g., violence risk assessment and management, individuals with sexual offending histories, how to work with probation and parole, familiarity with the statutes relevant to the forensic population) and then tasked UMMS to coordinate training sessions. These training sessions have been provided by UMMS faculty and by external experts identified by UMMS.

THE DESIGNATED FORENSIC PROFESSIONAL PROGRAM

The initial challenge, in 1986, was to ensure that psychologists assigned to conduct public-sector forensic evaluations would be forensically trained and practice consistently with the evolving standards in the field—but also in accordance with Massachusetts statutes and case law. In addition, since most courts had little experience with psychologists serving as forensic evaluators, DMH was intent on developing a rigorous process to ensure that the quality of the work produced would be high. To accomplish these goals, DMH and UMMS worked jointly to develop state regulations that would outline the broad requirements for psychologists to be forensically certified. An essential component of this process was the establishment by DMH of a DFP Committee to develop standards and oversee certification of forensic psychologists (and, a few years later, forensic psychiatrists as well). The committee is chaired by a UMMS Law and Psychiatry Program senior faculty member, with other members of the committee appointed by the Assistant Commissioner and drawn from experienced forensic psychologists and psychiatrists in the Commonwealth. (In 1999, a parallel committee, the Certified Juvenile Court Clinician Committee [CJCC] was established.) The details of the DFP process are described later; as may be seen, the CJCC process is similar to the original DFP process. The guidelines for the committees and the processes for certification were contained in state regulations.

Regulations

DMH regulations that specified requirements to apply for training and become a DFP, and the provisions for renewal and/or decertification, were developed. Over the past three decades there have been some modifications made to these regulations; for the purpose of clarity, this section focuses on the current regulations (104 CMR 33.03, 2019).

For psychologists, the qualifications to apply to become a DFP candidate include

a. licensure as a Health Service Provider Psychologist in Massachusetts (with special provisions for those licensed in other jurisdictions who may become provisional candidates pending obtaining licensure in Massachusetts);
b. 2,000 hours of clinical experience in a setting with adults with a mental illness or 1,000 hours of clinical experience in an inpatient psychiatric hospital that accepts adults with a mental illness (to ensure that the individual has sufficient expertise in diagnosis and assessment of individuals with severe and persistent mental illness, who constitute a large proportion of forensic evaluees);
c. is or will be employed in a setting in which he or she will be performing public-sector forensic evaluations as part of this position (to limit this credential to individuals actually working in the public sector);
d. letters of recommendation from at least two mental health professionals.

These requirements were designed to ensure that the psychologists undergoing specialized training in forensic psychology would have requisite foundational experience with individuals with severe and persistent mental illness who are the focus of the DMH's mandate. For psychiatrists, the requirements are similar—except instead of hours of experience with adult psychiatric patients, the requirement is to be board certified or board eligible in psychiatry. The rationale is that all psychiatrists have the requisite exposure to the relevant population as part of psychiatric residency, as opposed to psychologists who can become licensed without significant exposure to this population. In addition, as the program involves considerable resources from the state agency and the public university, training and certification was limited to those practitioners working in the public sector.

Once accepted as a candidate, the psychologist or psychiatrist is assigned a Forensic Mental Health Supervisor (FMHS). The supervisor is appointed from a pool of certified DFP psychologists and psychiatrists by the Assistant Commissioner, based on recommendation of the DFP Committee. There is a rigorous process involved in being appointed as a supervisor, including having at least 5 years of forensic mental health experience. Other requirements include

1. evidence of significant experience conducting forensic evaluations;
2. two letters of recommendation, one from a forensic clinician and one from a supervisee;
3. submission of two reports to be reviewed by the DFP Committee to determine quality of forensic work (at a higher level than required to be appointed a DFP); and
4. information from current work supervisors attesting to the quality and integrity of the candidate.

Training Model

The Massachusetts model is distinguished from most other state models by the investment in a very intensive mentoring and supervision process. In addition to attending didactic workshops (covering all types of evaluations that forensic evaluators conduct in the public sector), each trainee is assigned an FMHS whose role is to provide

instruction on the standards for performing evaluations; assistance in developing an understanding of basic concepts and laws relevant to forensic practice; instruction on how to identify and apply clinical data to psycho-legal questions; guidance in learning how to find and read relevant material and case law; feedback on written reports and consultation on providing testimony. (Massachusetts, 2019, p. 11)

The FMHS is not necessarily the trainee's administrative work supervisor; rather, the DMH committed to providing the necessary supervision using a cadre of experienced forensic evaluators. The supervisor and candidate develop a training plan that is approved by the DFP Committee. Candidates submit two sets of forensic reports to the committee. One set is sent about halfway through the training, so the candidate can get feedback from the committee on progress and areas for growth. The second set is sent when the candidate and supervisor think that the candidate has achieved the relevant competencies. These reports are reviewed by the committee, which decides whether the candidate demonstrates the necessary knowledge and skills to conduct these evaluations independently. If so, and if the candidate has passed the written examination, the committee recommends to the Assistant Commissioner that the individual be certified as a DFP.

The duties of the DFP Committee also include quality review to ensure that designated forensic psychologists and psychiatrists continue to practice in accord with expected standards. DMH has developed processes for identifying evaluators whose work has been flagged as potentially problematic. This can occur either through a Continuous Quality Improvement (CQI) process, involving periodic review of forensic reports, or if issues are identified by court personnel or supervisors. The reports are then sent to the DFP Committee for review. The Committee will review the reports and other relevant material (such as comments by those conducting the initial review and comments from the forensic evaluator) and determine if there are concerns about the evaluator's practice. The options for the committee, described in the DFP Procedures Manual (Massachusetts, 2019, p. 7), include

a. determining that no further action by the DFP Committee is needed;
b. providing feedback to the evaluator regarding issues raised by the review process;
c. providing formal consultation to the evaluator; or
d. determining that remedial supervision is required.

Consistent with the division of responsibility between the committee and DMH, the DFP Committee can recommend that remedial supervision be provided, but it is the Assistant Commissioner who makes the final decision and appoints a supervisor. If remediation is required, the assigned supervisor works with the candidate to develop a remediation plan to be submitted to the DFP Committee. Within one year, or whenever the assigned supervisor determines that adequate progress has been made, the evaluator will submit report samples to the DFP Committee for further review. At that point, the Committee recommends to the Assistant Commissioner either removal from remediation, continued remediation, or revocation of the DFP status.

The implementation of these policies and procedures requires communication and collaboration between UMMS and DMH. Over the three decades, there have been changes made to the procedures; these changes can be initially proposed either by the DFP Committee or by DMH. The roles of the committee and DMH are clearly delineated: the committee makes recommendations, but only the Assistant Commissioner has the authority to make final decisions about the appointment of DFPs and Supervisors, revocation of either of these statuses, and changes in policy and procedure.

Updates and Continuing Education

As there are advances in the field and new case law, it is essential that the content of the training be updated and mechanisms developed to allow practitioners to remain current in their knowledge and practices. Regarding the DFP training and certification, the written examination has required updating to reflect advances in practice as well as statutory and case law. The most recent update (2018) involved a significant restructuring of the examination into five content areas: CST, CR, violence risk assessment, practice issues (covering ethical standards as well as statutes, regulations, and case law), and evaluations for substance use disorder (as Massachusetts law, M.G.L. chapter 123, § 35 allows for commitment of individuals with a substance use disorder who are considered a risk of harm to self or others; this is the most frequent evaluation in court clinics; see Massachusetts, 2016). The examinations are scored by UMMS, with item analysis included. If certain items are answered incorrectly by most examinees, they will be reviewed by the DFP Committee to determine if they need to be reworded or if more attention needs to be devoted in training to those areas.

It is also important for practitioners to stay current on developments in the field. To accomplish this goal, UMMS developed a publication entitled "Expert Opinion" that was disseminated quarterly to all public-sector forensic practitioners and trainees. The publication included invited columns addressing interesting cases or topics, a column by the Assistant Commissioner of DMH with relevant news and perspectives, and updates on case law. This publication was supplanted in 2000 by the development of a website, which allowed for more flexibility (www.umassmed.edu/forensictraining). The website includes information about changes in certification procedures as well as updates on standards of practice. The website contains answers to frequently asked questions as well as other topics that are crucial to forensic practice such as guidelines for (1) informing evaluees of the limits of confidentiality and privilege, (2) writing a CR report when a defendant cannot provide an account of the alleged offense, and (3) dispositional recommendations.

UMMS faculty have played a very important role in this process, by (among other things) helping to translate case law into practice. For example, consider the landmark case of *Godinez v. Moran* (1993). In that case, the US Supreme Court ruled that standards for competence to plead guilty were the same as the standards for proceeding to trial because decision-making about defense pleas and strategy are an essential element of CST. In response, the DFP Committee amended the standards for writing trial competence reports to include a specific focus on decision-making in all cases. To further educate and inform practitioners, Dr. Grisso (who was then chair of the Committee) wrote a brief article about how to assess decision-making, which was disseminated on the website that UMMS developed in conjunction with DMH. In addition, the standardized training (Foundations) was modified to include this element.

A similar process was followed after the Massachusetts Supreme Judicial Court (SJC) handed down two significant rulings regarding the role of substance use in insanity defense cases (*Commonwealth v. Berry*, 2010; *Commonwealth v. DiPadova*, 2011). In these cases, the SJC ruled that a defendant who was both mentally ill and using substances at the time of the alleged offense could qualify for the insanity defense even if voluntary consumption of alcohol or other drugs activated or intensified the mental illness, unless "he knew (or should have known) that the consumption would have the effect of intensifying or exacerbating his mental condition" (*Commonwealth v. DiPadova*, p. 437). In addition, the court included language (in jury instructions) that "you should consider the question solely from the defendant's point of view, including her mental capacity and her past experience with drugs or alcohol" (*Commonwealth v. Berry*, p. 619, note 9). These cases added a significant issue for forensic evaluators, increasing the focus on whether the defendant knew at the time of the alleged offense of the effect that substance use could have on his or mental status. In response to these cases, changes were made in the Foundations training and in the report writing manual (chapter 123 section 15(b) Report Guidelines; Massachusetts, 2016). In addition, DMH asked Dr. Packer to provide a workshop to all court clinicians (video-recorded for ongoing use) addressing this issue as part of a refresher training.

Another element of continuing education involves the annual conference for all public-sector forensic professionals, coordinated by UMMS Law and Psychiatry and DMH. Each year DMH, in consultation with the leadership of the DFP and CJCC Committees, identifies topics that are considered relevant to practitioners in the field. UMMS then identifies presenters, drawing from national, local, and UMMS experts. This conference not only provides practitioners with updated knowledge and new developments in the field, but also is an opportunity to bring the forensic community together, contributing to a sense of shared purpose and allowing clinicians to exchange ideas and experiences.

Fellowship Programs

In addition to the training and certification of public-sector practitioners, the contract with DMH also included a provision for UMMS to develop a Forensic Psychology Postdoctoral Fellowship (now called a Residency) to provide a one year intensive training program. This program began in 1988, and in 1992 expanded to include a Forensic Psychiatry Fellowship. The fellowships include didactic seminars in Forensic Mental Health, a Landmark Cases seminar (review of national and local cases impacting forensic practice), clinical rotations in hospitals and court clinics, and a research component. An important advantage of siting these fellowships in the Medical School was that it allowed for fully integrated training of both forensic psychologists and psychiatrists. In addition, UMMS, by offering academic appointments, could attract highly qualified and experienced attorneys to oversee the legal aspects of the program and serve as a resource for the trainees by addressing legal issues that emerge. Furthermore, the Department of Psychiatry was also able to recruit highly respected forensic psychologists and psychiatrists to direct the fellowship programs. The advantage to DMH is that UMMS was able to draw highly qualified trainees from around the country, many of whom remained in Massachusetts and enriched the DMH forensic workforce.

An important element, as noted earlier, was the preexisting infrastructure of the Law and Psychiatry Program at UMMS. Although today forensic psychology is a recognized specialty by the American Psychological Association (APA), it was still a relatively new field in the mid-1980s. The ABFP (which certifies forensic psychology specialists) had been created as an independent board in 1978. Only in 1985 was it integrated into the American Board of Professional Psychology (ABPP). The fact that UMMS had several forensic psychiatrists on faculty provided an additional resource, at no additional cost, that augmented the didactic and training components of the newly developed forensic psychology postdoctoral program.

The UMMS forensic psychology postdoctoral fellowship has been recognized as the top-ranked program for the postdoctoral training of forensic psychologists (Helms, 2008), enhancing the reputation of the Medical School. The Forensic Psychiatry fellowship is accredited by the Accreditation Council for Graduate Medical Education (ACGME) following established standards. The Forensic Psychology Fellowship did not have guidance about standards from within its profession until 2008, following the APA's adoption of the Education and Training (E&T) Guidelines for Forensic Psychology (American Psychological Association, 2007). Rather, the elements of the program initially largely mirrored the psychiatry guidelines and were also informed by the professional literature. Since 2008, the program adheres to the APA E&T guidelines. The major elements of the fellowship programs include

1. rotations on forensic units or forensic hospitals, conducting pretrial evaluations of CST, CR, aid in sentencing evaluations, need for commitment, and prisoners in need of treatment;
2. conducting evaluations for violence risk assessment and management for patients on inpatient units with significant histories of violence;
3. conducting evaluations at court clinics, which include screening evaluations for CST and CR; evaluation for civil commitment; evaluation for commitment for substance use treatment;
4. other rotations, such as juvenile courts, assessment of sexually problematic behavior;
5. didactic seminar that covers the breadth of topics in Forensic Psychology and Psychiatry;
6. landmark cases seminar, covering relevant state cases, as well as national cases, consistent with the reading lists developed by the ABFP and the American Academy of Psychiatry and Law; and
7. the psychiatry fellowship including a treatment component, as this is a requirement of ACGME.

Measuring Effectiveness

Over the 32 years that the DFP program has been in existence, more than 200 forensic psychologists and psychiatrists have been certified through this process. (In addition, more than 100 psychologists and masters' level clinicians have been certified as Juvenile Court Clinicians.) Significantly, there are data to suggest that the training program has resulted in high-quality evaluations. As part of the development of a continuous quality improvement program by the DMH, three experienced forensic evaluators (two psychologists and one psychiatrist) reviewed a total of 122 CST reports and 102 CR reports. Based on consensus ratings, evaluators were rated as having obtained sufficient data for their conclusions in 89% of the CST reports and to have provided clear reasoning for their opinions in 93% of the reports reviewed. For CR reports, 80% were considered to have sufficient data, and 72% as having provided clear reasoning (Packer & Leavitt, 1998). These data contrast favorably with findings from other jurisdictions, as documented in the literature (e.g., Skeem & Golding, 1998; Warren, Murrie, Chauhan, & Morris, 2004). For instance, in the Skeem and Golding study, only about one-third of the CST reports were considered to have the conclusions clearly articulated based on the data. In the Warren et al. study, more than half of the CR reports reviewed lacked adequate data about the alleged offense. As lack of adequate training has been identified as a major factor in poor-quality forensic reports, the positive finding from Massachusetts attest to the effectiveness of the rigorous DFP training and certification program.

The forensic psychology postdoctoral program has also been very successful. In a survey of forensic psychologists by Helms (2008), the UMMS Forensic Psychology postdoctoral program was ranked first in terms of quality of postdoctoral training programs. In addition, the fellowship programs have served as a pipeline of highly qualified practitioners in the Massachusetts public sector. Over the first 31 years of the program, 42 psychology trainees (out of a total of 82) and 17 psychiatry trainees (out of a total of 41) have taken positions in the Massachusetts public sector, including a number in leadership roles. This has become even more relevant recently, as many of the evaluators who were trained early on have either retired or moved to other positions. The availability of highly trained fellows has provided an invaluable resource to a system that at times struggles to recruit forensic practitioners from other states. In addition, a number of the psychiatry trainees have taken positions as treating psychiatrists on forensic units. This has greatly enhanced the quality of care for forensic patients, as their treaters are well familiarized with the issues impacting these patients based on their legal status.

Contractual Arrangements

The arrangement between UMMS and DMH is set forth in a formal contract between the agencies. The contract stipulates the deliverables from UMMS and also contains a line-item budget based on cost reimbursement. This means that UMMS identifies actual costs, mostly salaries, but also including some nonpersonnel items such as travel, cost for attending workshops, and program support (e.g., office supplies, books for trainees), and is reimbursed for these actual expenses. The annual budget is currently about $450,000, of which about one-third reflects the cost (including tax, fringe, and overhead) of two forensic psychology residents (a third resident is covered through another contract). It should also be noted that the residents contribute to the system by conducting forensic evaluations that would otherwise be conducted by hiring additional salaried forensic psychologists thus effectively offsetting the cost. One of the biggest difficulties relates to budget issues. Any increase to the budget must be approved by DMH and can also be subject to legislative scrutiny. Thus, the budget has not been increased over many years. This can create difficulties as costs (such as salaries and fringe benefits) increase without commensurate increases in the funding from the DMH. Although creative workarounds have been used over the years (such as moving some faculty time to other contracts to reduce costs in this contract, or UMMS supplementing with other sources of funding), this has been a long-term challenge. For other programs starting up, it would be advisable to include a yearly cost of living increase in the contractual language. In addition, none of the faculty salaries was covered 100% by DMH. Rather, all of the faculty had other sources of income, either through other state contracts or external grant funding. The external grant funding has been an important source of revenue, bringing in more than $10 million in research grants across two decades. Although the contract funding was not used for the training program, it allowed UMMS to continue to support the faculty whose time was devoted to the DMH contract.

Another issue for this type of arrangement is buy-in from the leadership of both agencies. This program began with a clear sense of its mission as stated by the Assistant Commissioner, the Chair of the UMMS Department of Psychiatry, and the Director of the UMMS Law-Psychiatry Program. Over the past three decades, there have been multiple Assistant Commissioners and several different Department Chairs. Stability has been provided by the leadership of the training program—only two individuals, who have overlapped, and both of whom are still involved at some level with the program. However, as that is likely to change over the next few years, the challenge will be to ensure continuity of mission. To date, there has been clarity on all sides about the values, expectations, and desired outcomes. It will be important over time that all three leaders (program leader, chair, and Assistant Commissioner) communicate and develop mechanisms for resolving any differences.

What Has Worked

Both of the institutions have benefited from this collaboration. For DMH, the advantages have included

1. The establishment of clear standards for forensic mental health practice based on the ability of the academic institution to research the literature for best practice standards. In addition, UMMS has been able to draw on other resources, such as nationally recognized experts and its own faculty, to keep the field updated.

2. The academically run program has produced highly trained and competent evaluators who have enriched the public-sector workforce.
3. The involvement of the academic institution has enhanced the prestige of the DMH public-sector forensic system and has contributed to increased morale among the workforce.
4. The excellent reputation of the UMMS Forensic fellowship programs has attracted qualified professionals to Massachusetts.
5. DMH has been able to access UMMS faculty to consult on policy issues related to forensic mental health practice.

For the University, advantages include

1. DMH funding has allowed UMMS to grow their Law and Psychiatry faculty, bringing in more funding from external granting agencies.
2. The funding from DMH has allowed UMMS to attract highly qualified applicants to its training programs. The trainees have not only worked in the public sector, but have also taken faculty positions at UMMS, enhancing the psychiatry department's research, training, and clinical services.
3. UMMS has established a reputation as the premier forensic psychology postdoctoral training program in the country.
4. The success of the program has provided UMMS psychiatry department with opportunities to obtain other contracts from DMH.
5. UMMS faculty, through the close collaboration and involvement in all aspects of forensic mental health service in Massachusetts, have gained valuable knowledge and expertise that has contributed to their ability to establish standards for the broader field.

Lessons Learned

Several significant elements have contributed to the success of the DMH–UMMS collaboration. In addition, there are several caveats that other academic programs considering partnering with state agencies should consider. These include

1. Need for "buy-in" from leadership of the academic institution. In the case of UMMS, the commitment to public-sector work, in combination with the infrastructure of the Law and Psychiatry Program, created a positive environment for entering into the collaboration.
2. Need for clearly articulated—in writing—mission, goals, and deliverables. Although these were all stipulated in the contract, over time there was some slippage (such that the contract has not been updated in several years). In the case of the DMH–UMMS collaboration, this has not resulted in any problems as the leaderships of both agencies continue to be committed to the program and there has been stability in program

leadership. However, as this cannot always be guaranteed, it behooves both the state agency and the academic institution to ensure that there is updated written documentation.

3. Ongoing data collection to ensure that the program is meeting expectations. In Massachusetts, it is clear how the fellowship programs have provided valuable resources to the public sector in terms of trainees remaining in the system. The development of Continuous Quality Improvement (CQI) programs by DMH has provided a basis for assessing the quality of forensic reports.

4. There needs to be a thoughtful, long-term plan about budgetary issues. The major challenge for UMMS has been the lack of built-in increases for cost of living each year. Although creative ways have been found to cover costs, this is not something that can always be counted on. Rather, it would serve academic institutions well to include provisions for yearly increases in contractual arrangements. In addition, it is essential that faculty working on these collaborations have capacity for other sources of funding. It is unlikely that most state agencies can provide adequate funding for full-time faculty. Therefore, the faculty must have capacity to bring in other sources of funding through research grants, other service or training contracts, or direct clinical services.

5. This model worked well within a context of providing valuable education to prospective forensic psychologists and psychiatrists. It was important that clinicians viewed the certification as conferring status and value rather than as a restriction on practice. Much of this was specific to the model used in Massachusetts, which relied on state and vendor employees rather than private practitioners. However, it was also important that the field recognized that the standards were being developed and implemented by highly qualified and respected forensic professionals, based on evidence-based practice and consistent with national standards. The central role of UMMS as an academic center was an important factor in conferring credibility and status to the certification process.

CONCLUSION

The collaboration between UMMS and DMH has benefited both entities over a period of more than 30 years. DMH has benefited by developing a highly qualified workforce to provide forensic evaluations to the courts in Massachusetts. In addition, DMH has been able to draw on the resources of the UMMS Law and Psychiatry Program to provide additional training sessions and policy recommendations regarding issues such as violence risk assessment. UMMS has benefited by using DMH funding to attract qualified faculty who have brought in external grant and contract funding and who have made significant scholarly contributions, enhancing the reputation of the UMMS Psychiatry Department.

REFERENCES

104 CMR 33.03 (2019).

American Psychological Association. Education and Training Guidelines for Forensic Psychology (2007). https://www.apadivisions.org/division-41/education/guidelines.pdf

Commonwealth v. Berry, 457 Mass. 602 (2010).

Commonwealth v. DiPadova, 460 Mass. 424 (2011).

Fein, R. A., Appelbaum, K. L., Barnum, R., Baxter, P., Grisso, T., & Leavitt, N. (1991). The Designated Forensic Professional Program: A state government-university partnership to improve forensic mental health services. *Journal of Mental Health Administration, 18,* 223–230.

Godinez v. Moran, 509 U.S. 389 (1993).

Helms, J. (2008). *Forensic psychology program rankings.* Poster session presented at the American Psychology–Law Society annual conference, Jacksonville, FL.

Massachusetts. (2016). Chapter 123 section 15(b) Report Guidelines. https://www.mass.gov/files/documents/2016/07/vw/15b-report-writing-manual-cst-cr-appendix.pdf

Massachusetts. (2018). Designated Forensic Professional Procedures Manual. https://www.mass.gov/files/documents/2019/07/02/dfp-procedures-manual-revision-december-2018.pdf

Packer, I. K., & Leavitt, N. (1998). *Designing and implementing a quality assurance process for forensic evaluations.* Paper presented at American Psychology-Law Society Conference, Redondo Beach, CA.

Skeem, J., & Golding, S. (1998). Community examiners' evaluations of competence to stand trial: Common problems and suggestions for improvement. *Professional Psychology: Research and Practice, 29,* 357–367.

Warren, J. I., Murrie, D. C., Chauhan, P., & Morris, J. (2004). Opinion formation in evaluating sanity at the time of the offense: An examination of 5175 pre-trial evaluations. *Behavioral Sciences and the Law, 22,* 171–186. www.umassmed.edu/forensictraining

4

Establishing a Forensic Training Clinic

MARY ALICE CONROY ■

The Sam Houston State University (SHSU) Psychological Services Center (PSC) is the department training clinic for our doctoral program in clinical psychology. The doctoral program was established in 1998, with the overall purpose of providing broad-based training in clinical psychology, but with a special emphasis in forensic psychology. Using a scientist-practitioner model, we took the position that actual clinical forensic experience was critically important. We also had as a major element of our mission statement the provision of needed services to the community.

The need for training in forensic assessment was as clear in 1998 as it is today. Courts have increasingly called for services of assessment, treatment, and mental health consultation in the forensic arena (DeMatteo, Marczyk, Krauss, & Burl, 2009). Reports submitted to the courts were falling short of the quality needed (Heilbrun & Collins, 1995; see generally Melton et al., 2018). As is true today, the demand for high-quality forensic evaluations could not be met by the numbers of competent evaluators available (Heilbrun, Kelley, Koller, Giallella, & Peterson, 2013). There has been considerable debate in the field as to whether specific training in the forensic assessment area should be done at the graduate level or whether any specialization beyond broad and general clinical psychology should be done at the postdoctoral level (DeMatteo et al., 2009). Nonetheless, Otto and Heilbrun (2002) point out that many psychologists will find themselves being "accidental experts" to the court at some points in their careers. Some have argued that every psychologist should be prepared to be an expert witness (Bersoff et al., 1997; Fernandez, Davis, Conroy, & Boccaccini, 2009). While Packer (2008) strongly supported the need for specialty training at the postdoctoral level, he has also reported that forensic postdoctoral training slots are limited and have not kept pace with demand. Yet student demand for such training has been strong (Brigham, 1999).

Given the realities of the forensic world and gaps in services offered, it was determined by the clinical program faculty that the SHSU training clinic would devise a system to offer forensic assessments. To do so would require collaboration with the primary consumer of such services—the courts. The two basic purposes of this collaboration were clear. First and primary was to provide doctoral students with hands-on training in conducting forensic assessments. The second purpose was to provide the local courts with valuable services.

BEGINNINGS OF THE COLLABORATION

The collaboration began in 1999, soon after I accepted a faculty position to assist in developing the new doctoral program in clinical psychology with forensic emphasis. Members of the Texas State Educational Coordinating Board, the entity that approves new graduate programs in the state, were very clear that they saw no need for an additional general clinical doctoral program. Rather, they said that the forensic emphasis was key to the approval. SHSU was ideally positioned for interdisciplinary work in this area due to the university's large and well-regarded College of Criminal Justice.

It was suggested to me by the program faculty shortly after I arrived that I design a training clinic to support the developing doctoral program. I had just retired after 20 years with the US Bureau of Prisons, mostly spent in clinical and administrative positions in federal prison hospitals with major forensic missions. Although I had been heavily involved in forensic training of psychology interns and medical residents, I had almost no experience in outpatient settings or in the community mental health world. SHSU had a health center that served its student population but did not have anything resembling a training clinic and had no one with experience in providing community mental health services or any services in the forensic arena. I was left to my own devices and told to be creative.

Location

Among the first things to consider was the location of the university in Huntsville, Texas. This is a very rural area of southeast Texas, known primarily for being the center of the Texas state prison system. The closest university with a graduate training clinic in a psychology department was Texas A&M University (TAMU), in College Station, about an hour's drive from Huntsville. I quickly established a close working relationship with the TAMU training clinic director. It was from him that I learned the basics of operating a general clinical psychology training clinic. However, our program very much wanted to develop some subset of forensic services in which students could participate. Here our location served us well. To our south was the largest metropolitan area in the state (Houston) where forensic providers were relatively abundant. But to the north, east, and west were a number of small rural counties with almost no access to forensic assessment services. There was a definite need and very little competition.

Timing

In many ways, it was the ideal time to pilot a forensic training clinic. On a national level, a group was in the process of drafting a petition to have forensic psychology recognized as a discrete specialty area (Otto & Heilbrun, 2002). On the state level, considerable concern was being raised regarding the quality of mental health reports being submitted to the courts and the serious consequences that could result. A 501c(3) nonprofit organization called Capacity for Justice (https://www. capacityforjustice.org/) was actively lobbying state officials to improve the situation. A prominent state senator took up the cause and formed a task force to write a new statute regarding competence to stand trial evaluations. I was included on that taskforce along with five psychiatrists and four attorneys. The resulting statute (Texas Code of Criminal Procedure [2019] Title 1, Chapter 46B) set out very specific criteria for experts conducting these evaluations and also formed the basis for a subsequent statute regarding insanity evaluations (Texas Code of Criminal Procedure [2019], Title 1, Chapter 46C).

In addition to legislative movement in the areas of traditional criminal forensic evaluations, numerous states, including Texas, were considering ways to apply civil commitment procedures to certain sexual offenders. In 1999, Texas expanded the Health and Safety Code to include Title 11, Chapter 841, Civil Commitment of Sexually Violent Predators (Texas Health & Safety Code, 1999). Under this statute, forensic mental health evaluations were required to include the appraisal of psychopathy. This raised the possibility of another forensic experience for students in the area of violence risk assessment.

ESTABLISHING THE INITIAL OPERATION

In the initial organization of our forensic assessments, I relied on my experience in conducting and supervising forensic evaluations for the Bureau of Prisons as well as the experience of a colleague in the SHSU College of Criminal Justice who held both a PhD in clinical psychology and a law degree (JD) and who was previously a Texas law enforcement officer. No prior collaborations of this nature in Texas had been established, so we were building from the ground up. We were limited by the expertise of available supervisors and time available. This meant limiting our assessments to the criminal courts, as is now somewhat typical of forensic operations at the graduate level (Heilbrun et al., 2013). We expanded slightly to include sexually violent predator evaluations that are considered civil in nature.

Initial Marketing

Outreach to the courts was first done primarily by a series of letters to local judges and presentations at local bar association meetings. Sexually violent predator evaluations have always been performed under contract with the administration of the Texas Department of Criminal Justice (TDCJ), conveniently housed in Huntsville, so they were approached as well. Flyers and local newspaper articles describing the newly opened PSC, including our forensic operations, were also circulated throughout the Huntsville area.

Workshop Presentations

In an additional effort at outreach, our faculty offered several workshops to the community at large aimed at training and honing the skills of forensic evaluators. Our campus had ample resources for holding such events, as well as mechanisms for offering continuing education credit. These were generally successful. When the Capacity for Justice organization became aware of our community training efforts, they invited us to join them in presenting such workshops statewide. This collaboration has expanded and continues to this day, and it now includes training for attorneys and medical providers.

THE PARTICIPANTS

The PSC opened to the public in 1999 and offered its first forensic services in 2000. The five clinical psychologists on the doctoral program faculty were generally expected to supervise work performed by students at the PSC, with occasional support from other clinical faculty who volunteered to teach practicum classes. Initially, I was the only supervisor who had the specific qualifications and experience to supervise students in the forensic arena. In 2000, we received 11 court orders for forensic assessments, so this was quite doable. However, our referrals subsequently expanded beyond what anyone had expected. Between 2001 and 2005, we completed 50 competence to stand trial evaluations and 27 sanity evaluations. Over the next 5 years, from 2005 to 2010, our volume of forensic services increased by more than 100%. It became clear that one supervisor could not adequately manage this task. In 2007, we hired a clinical staff psychologist whose duties were only to supervise students in clinical and forensic work. In 2008, a Spanish-speaking psychologist with forensic experience joined our faculty. Over the next decade, demand for forensic assessments increased dramatically, and, in 2014, a second staff clinician was brought on to provide primarily forensic supervision. Between the two primary forensic supervisors in 2018, 154 forensic assessments were completed for the courts—14 times the number completed during our first year. The second staff psychologist was responsible for regular clinical supervision as well as supervision of general juvenile evaluations, referred either by the court or by a probation department.

All of our doctoral students have the opportunity to participate in assessments for the courts. Looking at records of students who graduated from our program between 2007 and 2018, the number of evaluations per student during their time on campus varied from 1 to 41. The average number of forensic evaluations students complete while in residence at SHSU is 13.

WHO IS SERVED?

During our first year of offering forensic evaluations to the courts, we served primarily four local judges in our home county, which has a population of approximately 70,000 people. Over the past 3 years, we have provided evaluations for 35 judges in 20 counties—that is 8% of the counties in the State of Texas. Counties served ranged from relatively large and urban (e.g., Montgomery County has a population of approximately 556,000 and is served by seven district and five county courts) to small and rural (e.g., Trinity County has a population of approximately 14,000 and is served by a visiting judge).

Jail-Based Services

Serendipitously, our forensic operation also provides service to county correctional facilities within reasonable driving distance. This is because jails in this area have been pushed to capacity housing persons with serious mental illness who are waiting for their cases to proceed or to be referred for hospitalization. If we can provide evaluations quickly, the process can be moved along. Student clinicians accompany the forensic supervisor to nine jails on a regular basis, giving our students the experience of providing services in a correctional environment. Several distant facilities have agreed to transport inmates to our clinic for forensic evaluations.

Consultation

Our clinic has put strong emphasis on doctoral-level psychology trainees mastering consultation skills. Forensic evaluations are almost always a form of consultation to the courts or to attorneys. In addition, our faculty have provided training to numerous law enforcement agencies over the years regarding working with persons suffering from serious mental illness. More recently we have sought opportunities to include our students in these efforts. Specifically, in conjunction with the National Institute of Corrections (NIC), we participated in creating training materials for a statewide effort to train jail mental health officers. Our clinic also designed a workshop for police departments in the area to enhance their skills in dealing with persons who present challenges due to mental illness. Most recently, we have been invited by the Chief of Forensic Medicine for the Texas state hospital system to collaborate with them in providing training in forensic assessment for state hospital evaluators and other personnel.

HOW THE OPERATION FUNCTIONS

Toward the end of their first year in the program students go through a period of preparation before participating fully in forensic evaluations. I am then responsible for seeing that specific procedures are followed.

Class Preparation

Students are first introduced to forensic assessments during their third semester of graduate school. During that time, they take an initial practicum class that mainly involves practicing clinical interviewing skills during mock interviews. There is also an observation requirement that can be fulfilled by observing the supervisor and a student clinician conducting forensic evaluations. This is limited to one observer per session, but our volume is such that every student in the class has several opportunities to observe. The following semester students begin a year-long course in forensic assessment. About midway through this course, students may begin full participation in these evaluations. From that time on, students may volunteer for forensic evaluations throughout their time on campus. There has never been a shortage of volunteers.

The Court Order

Forensic evaluations are conducted almost exclusively under court order. This is advantageous in that it generally means we share the judge's immunity from civil suit, and disclosure/notification of purpose rather than fully informed consent is required with the examinee (Heilbrun, Grisso, & Goldstein, 2009). We occasionally receive orders written ex parte for assistance to the defense, but the work is still done by court order. Types of evaluations conducted, from most to least common, include competence to stand trial, sanity at the time of the offense, juvenile fitness to proceed and responsibility for conduct, violence risk assessment, mitigation, certification/waiver to adult court, and competence for execution. On rare occasions, we also evaluate various other competencies (e.g., competence to sign a contract, competence for adoption, competence to consent to sexual activity).

The Process

Once a court order is received, a student clinician is selected along with a time slot for the forensic interview. If not included with the order, the prosecutor is contacted and appropriate offense information is requested. If the examinee is incarcerated, the responsible correctional personnel are contacted to reserve confidential space for the evaluation. The defense attorney is notified of the time of the evaluation, and, if the examinee is in the community, this attorney is responsible for ensuring the person appears at the PSC at the appointed time. The defense attorney is generally welcome to attend the evaluation with an understanding that he or she remains out of the examinee's line of vision and does not interrupt the interview. However, attorneys rarely take advantage of this opportunity. The defense attorney is also asked to provide any available records, particularly mental health records. Texas statutes regarding competence and sanity evaluations require that the parties (both defense and prosecution) provide specific records to the appointed expert (Texas Code of Criminal Procedure, Title 1, Chapter 46B; Texas Code of Criminal Procedure, Title 1, Chapter 46C).

Both the student clinician and the supervisor review all records received. The interview is conducted jointly with student and supervisor. This appears to be similar to the procedure used by forensic evaluators at Drexel University (Heilbrun et al., 2013). Collateral interviews may be conducted as needed, often including interviews with jail staff. Once all data are assembled, the student clinician constructs an initial draft of the forensic report. It is then edited liberally by the responsible supervisor and signed by both student and supervisor. The edited document is then returned to the student and discussed. If court testimony is required on any case, this is done by the supervisor, and students are welcome to attend. Students are also welcome to participate in pretrial conferences with attorneys. It should be noted that, over many years, subpoenas to court have been relatively rare, perhaps one to two per year. Recently, cases have become more numerous and more complex, resulting in approximately a five-fold increase in the call for court testimony. This has provided students more opportunity to observe court testimony but has resulted in increased demands on supervisor time.

MOST EFFECTIVE EXPECTATIONS AND AGREEMENTS

From the outset, we realized we would need to address concerns of our students, our supervisors, the courts, and correctional personnel.

Student Concerns

Concerns have been frequently voiced to me by forensic practitioners regarding the inclusion of students in these evaluations, particularly if students are to function as co-participants. Evaluators question whether courts or attorneys will object to such an arrangement, whether students will be subpoenaed to provide expert testimony, or whether this may, in fact, violate various statutes requiring experts to be licensed or otherwise credentialed. Hedge and Brodsky (2013) discuss these specific issues as potentially causing attorneys concern. However, in my almost 20 years of experience providing these assessments in Texas—or, for that matter, my 20 years of using this model with interns in the Bureau of Prisons—this has never been an issue: consumers simply need to be informed that this is standard practice in the organization. Texas courts seeking our services are aware of the inclusion of students and the role played by those students. Under special circumstances, such as an evaluation conducted on Death Row, we will request that the court order specify that a student assistant will be included so that their admission to the facility will not be challenged. Judges with whom I have spoken often compare it to the system used by courts themselves, where law clerks may research and draft court opinions but everyone knows who is the responsible party. Since our opening of the forensic operation in 2000, the PSC has never had a student clinician called to court to provide expert testimony. Only twice in my federal career can I recall this happening: once when the court wanted specific testimony on the administration of psychological tests and once when a defendant was contending that I had never personally spoken with her. I had no concerns about either appearance. Texas statutes regarding competence to stand trial and sanity at the time of the offense have very specific requirements about an appointed expert's qualifications (Texas Code of Criminal Procedure, Title 1, Chapter 46B; Texas Code of Criminal Procedure, Title 1, Chapter 46C). In addition to state licensure, these include certain advanced training requirements that must be updated on an annual basis. The judiciary here has always understood that these requirements apply to the supervisor and not the student assistant. The decisions regarding the conduct of the evaluation, the data to be included, and the ultimate issue opinion are all those of the supervisor.

Working for the Judge

It has proved very effective to operate the forensic evaluation system by court order. This serves to reduce many issues of bias and the "allegiance effect" that research suggests may cause evaluators to tilt data in the direction of the party who hires them (Murrie, Boccaccini, Guarnera, & Rufino, 2013). It also reduces the requirement from formal informed consent to disclosure. This is particularly advantageous when the examinee is acutely psychotic and likely not competent to give informed consent. Obtaining some type of substitute consent can often result in delays and the subsequent resetting of court hearings. Finally, the court order often opens the door to speaking with both attorneys as well as collateral sources in pursuit of necessary information.

Working in a Correctional Environment

Expanding our services to include jail-based evaluations, even those involving some travel, has proved advantageous. When we conduct evaluations of examinees in the community, we find that approximately 20% of them fail to appear as scheduled. Although an incarcerated individual may, on very rare occasions, refuse to speak with us, they will be available for observation. This can be particularly important with individuals who are severely regressed, such as those creating severe disruption with no apparent rational motive or whose hygiene is severely deteriorating, even playing with their own excrement. This also allows students the experience of various jail environments. Jail staff of all types are often excellent informants regarding persons they have interacted with over time. Records provided, both medical and correctional, can paint an important picture of the individual's pattern of functioning. Students quickly learn the value of long-term relationships with correctional personnel and how best to interact with them. In addition, these relationships have furthered our efforts and credibility to provide consultation and training for jail personnel who are dealing with individuals with mental health problems.

Judicial Relationships

Relationships with judges and attorneys can have a positive impact well beyond conducting individual forensic assessments. For example, significant numbers of faculty in our department conduct research projects related to law enforcement or the judiciary. Officers of the court have been most helpful to those conducting jury research or surveys of various players in the legal system. Finally, judges and attorneys who have expressed their appreciation for our services have impressed the senior leadership in our university, which has resulted in increased university support for our forensic mission.

PROBLEMS ADDRESSED

Steps had to be taken to reduce the growing workload for supervisors. These included altering the fee schedule, eliminating SVP evaluations, and insisting on specific levels of cooperation from attorneys.

The Ever-Increasing Workload

A major oversight at the onset of this operation was not anticipating the number of evaluations that might be involved. In 2000, it was extremely rare for training facilities to include graduate students in actual forensic evaluations so there were no models to go by. In addition, with the greater metropolitan Houston area directly to our south, it seemed that this region might have been overrun with qualified forensic evaluators. We were very uncertain what, if any, forensic business would come to us. That said, we simply let courts in our immediate area know that we were open to providing forensic evaluations. Given the 11 court orders we received during our first year, this appeared very manageable. However, demand for our services quickly escalated. From 2001 to 2005, the PSC conducted 54 forensic evaluations. During the period 2006–2010, the total number of evaluations reached 283, which represents a significant increase over the previous 5-year period. Fast forward to the most recent 5 years (2015–2019, projecting through the remainder of 2019)—we will have conducted a total of 752 evaluations. This represents an enormous increase relative to the initial period. Our graduate students are delighted with the opportunity to engage in many evaluations. However, even with the addition of two forensically qualified supervisors, this rate of increase (if it continues) will soon be unsustainable. With hindsight, we should have considered capping the overall number of court orders we would accept or further circumscribing the area of Texas we were willing to serve.

Revising Our Forensic Fee Schedule

The mission of our clinic overall was to serve poor and underserved populations at low cost. We were clear in our communication with senior university leadership that our mission was training for our students and service to the community— and *not* generating significant amounts of revenue. As such, we adopted a generous sliding scale for our regular clinical services and very low fixed rates for our forensic services. Initially we established rates for various types of forensic assessments of between $250 and $350. Rates have been raised twice since that time and are now between $500 and $600, with exceptions made for evaluations requiring unusually extensive record reviews. However, again in hindsight, we should have begun with considerably higher fees and raised them more aggressively. In the long run, this would probably have raised more funds for our operation while reducing the number of evaluations ordered.

All of our forensic assessments are conducted simply in response to court order, including ex parte orders instructing us to work directly with the defense. We have no contracts with any individual courts. The fee schedule was communicated to all courts ordering services. In establishing our initial fee schedule, it became clear that the usual hourly rate charged by a single practitioner was not feasible. Would we be considering supervisor hours, student hours, case complexity, or travel time? We therefore began with simple, flat fees. If a single report was required (e.g., competence to stand trial) there was one fee, if two reports were required (e.g., competence to stand trial and legal sanity) there was a higher fee, and if we traveled to a facility outside of our county, a specific travel fee was added. Court testimony is provided by the supervisor, so a reasonable hourly fee ($85/ hour) is charged, but one still below what the person would charge as a private practitioner. Over our 20 years of operation, we have raised fees twice. This was done simply by writing to all of the judges who utilize our services and enclosing the new fee schedule. The courts seem to realize that our fees are relatively low overall because we are a training clinic, and there has never been a complaint when fees were raised.

Abandoning Sexually Violent Predator Evaluations

Early in our clinic development, we decided to contract with the TDCJ to conduct evaluations of sexual offenders who were due to be released and were being considered for civil commitment as Sexually Violent Predators. Texas had the first statute allowing only for outpatient commitment for these individuals, which was initially hailed as progressive and appeared to provide for a least restrictive environment. Such evaluations gave students the chance to conduct formal violence risk assessments. In addition, the Texas SVP statute specifically requires the expert to evaluate psychopathy, and this provided the opportunity for student training and experience in use of the Psychopathy Checklist-Revised (PCL-R). However, I had concerns regarding the structure of the statute itself and the consequences to those evaluated. The Texas SVP statute specifically requires evaluators to assess for a "behavioral abnormality," with no clear definition of what this meant and no known relationship to a clinical diagnosis or concept. TDCJ took the position that, since no court petition had been filed at the time of the evaluation, the offender had no right to counsel despite the fact that the evaluation would be used in court once a petition for commitment had been filed. As time went on, we consulted with the Council in charge of overseeing the outpatient program. It became increasingly clear that persons released to these outpatient conditions were subject to severe conditions that often impeded them from securing employment, living with their families, or securing suitable housing in some areas that were not restricted. We were also informed that 97 specific conditions were automatically imposed on these individuals, making it highly likely that they would fail to comply in some way and be returned to prison. For example, they were prohibited from associating with children—including their own family members—even if their offense had nothing to do with children. After several years, much soul-searching, and after supervising 140 SVP evaluations for TDCJ, I made the decision to withdraw from the contract for these reasons.

Relationships with Attorneys

Defense attorneys are always notified in writing of pending evaluations, and records, specified in statute, are requested from them. However, the majority of appointed attorneys make little or no effort to comply. This can often be a significant handicap to conducting a thorough evaluation. It would have been wise to set up specific procedures with the courts to ensure that important records are provided.

An additional problem with some attorneys occurs when examinees are on bond in the community. It then becomes the responsibility of the attorney to notify the examinee of the evaluation and its importance and to ensure that the person can attend. However, some attorneys did not do this, resulting in considerable wasted evaluator time. For the past 2 years, a caveat has been added to our attorney notification letters saying, "Given our heavy workload for the courts, should this individual fail to appear for this appointment, it cannot be rescheduled and you will need to seek another evaluator." Although some exceptions are made (e.g., the individual has just been hospitalized), this warning has reduced missed appointments.

MAJOR CHANGES SINCE THE BEGINNING

Over the 20 years of providing forensic services through our training clinic, a number of significant changes have been made.

Evaluations in Spanish

One major expansion has been the offering of forensic services in Spanish. This is a language skill in high demand in this geographic area. Since acquiring the Spanish-speaking forensic supervisor in 2008, we have been very conscious of the need to recruit Spanish-speaking students as part of our cohorts. During the past year, this has also led us to beginning offering immigration court services. Several of our faculty have had special training in this regard. We are now actively involved in conducting special hardship evaluations for these courts. Time and resources allowing, we remain open to other types of work with immigration courts.

Student Opportunities for Consultation

Over the past 5 years, we have consciously sought opportunities for our students to engage with us in forensic consultation beyond simply providing assessments and opinions to the courts. We were aware that another university in our geographic area, the University of Houston, had provided consultation on family law issues. Specifically, the University of Houston Center for Forensic Psychology has a model for providing consultation in this arena to attorneys throughout the state and beyond (http://www.uh.edu/class/psychology/clinical-psych/research/forensic/expert-services/). We invested our energies in the criminal arena, beginning with law enforcement training and expanding to the training of forensic evaluators for our state hospital system. This focus has been appreciated by our students because it has offered them some unique and valuable experiences.

The first statewide training for forensic examiners in the Texas state hospital system was conducted on September 4, 2019. We met at a central location in

Austin, Texas, where one of our large state facilities is located. Staff from that facility attended in person while all of the other state hospital staffs engaged in forensic work attended by teleconference. The event was deemed successful by the state administrators, and it was determined that this would be at least an annual event going forward. However, the real question, as always, is whether such training and consultation affects the evaluations that are conducted and the reports that are written. Being very aware of this, we agreed to assist in a long-term program evaluation effort.

Research

Given our strong forensic emphasis, many of our students concentrate their research in the forensic arena. As we enter our twentieth year of operations, the PSC retains large amounts of forensic data. In the early years of operation, we realized that we were in an excellent position to encourage research on site. However, we were a relatively small program and tended to prioritize setting up a service plan, assuring that supervision was in place, and providing quality assessments that the community was requesting. In recent years, however, we have been more actively promoting research opportunities. One problem is that almost all of our evaluations have been conducted by the same small group of supervisors. Therefore, research involving the comparison of forensic reports is limited. Nonetheless, researchers are encouraged to examine forensic assessments in terms of range of psychopathology, examinee demographic differences, changes over time, bases on which findings are made, and so forth. All research in our department is reviewed by an institutional review board (IRB). Students in our program have been granted clinical privileges at the PSC, giving them full access to our file data, and our IRB has been supportive of this approach. Going forward we hope to make up for research opportunities missed.

CONTRACTUAL AND FINANCIAL ARRANGEMENTS

Almost all invoices are sent directly to the court by one of my administrative assistants, along with the report. In the case of ex parte orders, this material goes to the attorney with the understanding that they will pass on the expense statement. The administrative staff are responsible for informing me of any problems with the billing and collection process. I am not aware of any case for which we have not received payment, nor of any case in which the court attempted to reduce the fee. Data have remained steady over the years indicating that although forensic evaluations are only 25% of the clinic's activities, they provide about 40% of the clinic's annual income. In other words, the forensic income helps to underwrite the clinical services made available to our low-income population.

Unlike our evaluations for the courts, our consulting/training services all involve formal contracts. These are generally negotiated by us and then reviewed by the legal departments of both agencies. The roles played by graduate students and those played by licensed supervisors are clearly delineated.

All fees collected for forensic work go directly to the clinic and are used to support student training at our discretion. No "indirect costs" are taken by the university. These monies are typically invested in testing equipment, books and manuals, honoraria paid to invited speakers, and student travel to conferences or special training opportunities, and to support travel to internship interviews. We have seen a steady increase in income from forensic services over the years. In our first year of operation, our total collected from forensic work was $2,750. In 2018, this figure was $81,100.

MEASURING EFFECTIVENESS

In my early years doing forensic evaluations for the US Bureau of Prisons, a number of us attempted to obtain feedback on these efforts from the courts we served. However, our efforts were generally unsuccessful. Requests for feedback produced a very low rate of return and included almost no useful, specific information. After 20 years of conducting/supervising federal court-ordered evaluations and 20 years of conducting/supervising such evaluations for the State of Texas, I have concluded that the best measures of consumer satisfaction revolve around four basic questions:

- How frequently are complaints raised?
- To what extent has the operation grown over time?
- Do consumers typically return for additional services?
- How frequently are we called to court to defend our reports?

Complaints

Over the past 20 years, several attorneys have challenged our analyses and opinions. That is the nature of the forensic beast. However, no complaints from any court, orally or in written form, have ever been received. No licensing board complaints nor complaints to any professional ethics board have ever been filed regarding our forensic work. No court has ever questioned the inclusion of students in our forensic assessments.

Demand for Forensic Services

The demand for our forensic work has steadily increased from 11 forensic assessments in our first year to 154 in 2018. Over the past 2 years, it has become necessary to decline some evaluations.

Looking at data from the 41 judges who have sent us court orders over the past 5 years, numbers of orders from individual judges range from 1 to 75 with a mean of 17. We clearly have a significant number of judges who refer cases to us on a regular basis. Judges with the smallest numbers (i.e., less than 5) are those from relatively small counties with fewer defendants and, therefore, less need for services.

Court Testimony

I have always been told by colleagues—and I have always told my students—that the better quality report one produces the less likely it is that the evaluator will be called to court to defend it. We are all aware that the vast majority of criminal cases are resolved through negotiated plea, without going to trial. For the first 18 years of our forensic operations, I was never called to court more than twice, and, in many years, I made no court appearances. This past year brought a slight increase in these numbers with eight court appearances between the two primary forensic supervisors. Given the increasing volume of evaluations, however, these numbers are still reasonably low.

Proximal Student Outcomes

Given that our mission is the training of doctoral students, we are especially concerned about the positive and potentially negative effects the forensic emphasis may have on them and their careers. Two proximal issues have potential negative effects. One issue often noted by students entering the program is a fear that they will be pulled into court and put on the witness stand to testify about matters for which they lack credentials, experience, and expertise. Supervisors from other institutions have also given this as the reason they would never allow student involvement in forensic assessments. This has never happened during our 20 years of operation. Occasionally, in very high-profile cases, initial subpoenas will be served on a large number of possible witnesses, and this has caused students high anxiety. As the actual hearing or trial came into focus, students have been invariably removed from the list.

A second issue of concern for students is estimating and balancing time commitments. In the forensic arena, it is often impossible to know at the onset the amount of collateral records needing review, the number of collateral interviews required, or even whether the interview of the defendant can be accomplished in a single session. Because our students are eager to volunteer for forensic assessments, I have found it necessary to carefully monitor student workloads.

Distal Outcomes for Students

More distal outcomes relating to student career achievements are critical in evaluating the overall success of any program. Although it is not possible to clearly link student training and experience in forensic assessment to overall outcomes, we believe there is an association. Since receiving our initial accreditation from the American Psychological Association (APA) in 2006, all of our students have matched with APA accredited internships. This included matching during the lean years when match rates were low enough nationwide to cause grave uncertainty. Virtually all of our graduates are employed or in practice. Annual follow-up surveys suggest that most of them are utilizing the forensic skills they initially acquired at SHSU. We now have 10 graduates who are board certified by the American Board of Professional Psychology (nine in forensic psychology and one in clinical neuropsychology). One of our graduates is currently serving on the board of the American Board of Forensic Psychology.

Accreditation

Accreditation by the APA Commission on Accreditation (CoA) is a critical issue for any clinical psychology doctoral program. When we first approached the CoA, we received a somewhat negative response, being told that training in forensic psychology was not a recognized area of doctoral-level clinical training. However, following some revision to our initial self-study, saying we were a clinical psychology doctoral program with forensic emphasis, we were granted a site visit in 2006 that resulted in full accreditation. We have since been reaccredited twice, most recently in 2018 for a full 10 years. In 2018, we found that forensic training significantly helped our accreditation efforts in the areas of consultation and diversity. The CoA seemed to agree that all of our forensic assessment work was consultation and provided students opportunities to consult both with officers · of the court and with law enforcement. In terms of diversity, it was clear that, through forensic assessments, our students had experience with a great variety of populations and saw a very broad spectrum of psychopathology.

SERVICES DELIVERED AND OTHER PRODUCTS

Over our 20 years of operation, the PSC has provided forensic assessment services to the court, as well as consultation and training to organizations involved with the legal system.

Forensic Assessment

As of August 2019, the SHSU clinical psychology doctoral program had awarded doctoral degrees to 104 individuals. In our most recent collation of 10-year outcome data, 96% of our graduates have become licensed. Going forward, with the blessing of our university hierarchy, we are planning to accept 7–8 students into the program annually. Although some of our students participate in only a small number of forensic assessments, most are involved in between 15 and 20 while in graduate school. Given what we know from follow-up with our students, these individuals are likely to continue conducting or supervising forensic evaluations as a major part of their careers.

Consultation and Training

Providing consultation and training to both the law enforcement community and to community mental health evaluators has become a more prominent part of our program in recent years. As such, we have created training materials for a variety of settings and groups. These have included a number of video examples of various forensic interviews that have been sanitized and role-played by our students. We make these materials available to others who may want to use them. We have also partnered with a detention center to create video clips of significant psychopathology.

LESSONS LEARNED

The SHSU Psychological Services Center opened in 1999, with a plan for offering the traditional clinical assessment and intervention services to the public along with offering forensic assessment services to the courts. At that time, I knew of no models of graduate school training clinics offering forensic services. My vision was that the forensic component would be limited. I was not even certain that, as a training clinic, we would attract much business from the courts.

Providing Supervision

Properly supervising court-ordered evaluations is heavily time-consuming, requiring that the supervisor be present and responsible for the entire procedure. This means it is advisable that a clinic offering forensic services have a number of well-qualified supervisors to share the workload. Given the demands, a system should be put in place to provide adequate compensation to these individuals, whether it be monetary or course release time. Currently, SHSU forensic supervisors simply have this supervision as part of their job descriptions. Legal consultation should also be readily available.

Contractual Relationships with Courts

The simplest and often legally least problematic way to receive forensic work is by court order. This has worked well for us. However, there also needs to be a contract with each court one intends to serve limiting the number of evaluations that will be accepted over any given time period. By not doing this, we found ourselves overwhelmed with forensic work. Although our students are delighted with the many opportunities, supervisors are often badly overextended. Once courts become accustomed to simply sending orders, it is a very difficult system to change. Contracts also need to clearly delineate the responsibilities of the parties. Texas law on competence and sanity evaluations is very clear as to what the court, the defense, and the prosecutor must provide. However, it is sometimes the case that we do not receive relevant information, whatever the statute may specify. For example, prosecutors are to provide to the expert all available offense information and defense attorneys are to provide any relevant mental health information. In each new county we serve, we find ourselves explaining this to the parties. However, when an order is signed, prosecutors and defense attorneys receive a copy; this should immediately trigger them to provide the expert with the required information. (Unfortunately, it does not.) Also, I discovered to my surprise that orders often did not specify the whereabouts of the defendant. Ideally, a contractual arrangement should put the responsibility on the defense attorney to make the examinee available for the forensic appointment if the individual is not incarcerated.

Contracts can also clearly establish what a court order needs to contain. I have a number of sample court orders that include language about agencies and practitioners providing any and all relevant records to the forensic evaluator. Such orders greatly reduce the time involved in collecting collateral information. They also give important sources, such as jail staff, permission to share data with evaluators.

Financial Arrangements

Students in our program receive no direct compensation for participating in forensic assessments. However, they seek these assessments with some eagerness due to the role of this experience in securing preferred internships. They also realize that money from forensic assessment fees is used for important purposes, such as funding travel expenses to internship interviews.

To have students fully participating in forensic work, I would strongly encourage setting flat fees rather than attempting hourly rates. However, it is important to find out the going rate for such work in a particular location. It is acceptable for a training clinic to charge rates that are somewhat lower than the community standard. However, if prices are initially set too low, there may well be complaints from community practitioners that they are being undercut, particularly if the clinic is part of a state agency. In addition, if rates are too low, services may seem too attractive, resulting in more business than can reasonably be managed.

Another financial issue is the cost of travel. Many criminal defendants are in jail. There are several advantages to conducting evaluations in a jail setting. In our clinic, we travel regularly to nine different detention centers, all of them operating somewhat differently. This gives a student seriously interested in a forensic career important experiences. It also reduces the need for shackles during an evaluation. Traveling to the jail generally ensures that the defendant will be there and available. It also gives the evaluation team the opportunity to interview various members of the jail staff. Another option is to insist that the examinee be brought to the clinic. However, this may be problematic in some locations, plus the opportunity for staff interviews is lost. Also, depending on the location and setting of the clinic, armed officers sitting in the hallways might not be desirable. It also costs the county more to send a deputy and a car, and to keep that deputy off-site for the duration of the evaluation. Since we do travel to jails, our fee schedule includes an extra $100 if we have to travel outside of Walker County.

Data Maintenance

At the onset of establishing a forensic section of a training clinic, a careful plan should be made for how data on these evaluations will be organized in a user-friendly manner. It is likely that in a number of years the clinic will have a great deal of archival data of value to the forensic researcher. While much of this can be maintained electronically, paper data are still apt to be received from outside sources. Unfortunately, we began our forensic record system simply by having files organized in alphabetical order. From my current perspective, I realize how valuable it would be to have an electronic system whereby files could contain (and hence be searched by) variables such as year of the case, age of the defendant, crime, psychopathology, instruments used, ultimate issue opinions, county, and a host of other intriguing categories. With hindsight, I would say this might have inspired a great deal more forensic research in our clinic.

Policies

Students, as well as clerical staff, need policies on important issues that differentiate forensic work from other clinical endeavors. For example, who owns the record? In regular clinical work, the client is the person who is being examined, and that person is entitled to receive or release their own record. In the case of a forensic assessment, the "client" is likely to be either the judge or an attorney, and the examinee is not entitled to have or release that record.

Some forensic evaluators routinely record their interviews. If not, they are likely to take copious contemporaneous notes. These need to be preserved. Are they to be kept separately, or are they part of the defendant's file?

Informed consent documents used for general clinical clients are not likely to be appropriate for a forensic evaluation. If evaluations are court-ordered, they are likely to require disclosure/notification rather than informed consent. As in the case of Texas, professional boards in many jurisdictions have very specific rules about what such notification must contain.

There needs to be a specific protocol to be followed when an investigator arrives with a subpoena for a person or a record. And, depending on the particular type of forensic work a clinic does, there may be other policy needs.

CONCLUSION

If done well, a forensic arm to a training clinic can have great value to students, the community, and the profession. Estimates are that more than 60,000 compe-tence for trial evaluations are ordered in the United States each year (Melton et al., 2018)—and that is just one kind of forensic evaluation. Numbers alone attest to the fact that the majority of this work is not done by forensic specialists who have completed forensic postdoctoral training and achieved board certification. This experience at the graduate level can provide training yielding specific specialized skills in early-career psychologists. It may also inspire some to seek further spe-cialized expertise. In addition, a training clinic, well run and well conceptualized, can provide invaluable service to the judicial community. Particularly in isolated, rural areas, qualified forensic evaluators may be at a premium. Here is an oppor-tunity to fill that gap.

REFERENCES

Bersoff, D. N., Goodman-Delahunty, J., Grisso, T. Hans, V., Poythres, N. G., & Roesch, R. (1997). Training in law and psychology: Models from the Villanova Conference. *American Psychologist, 52*, 1301–1310. doi:1997-43865-00310.1037/0003-066X.52.12.1301

Brigham. J. C. (1999). What is forensic psychology, anyway? *Law and Human Behavior, 23*, 273–298. doi:1999-03609-00110. 1023/A 1022304414537

DeMatteo, D., Marczyk, K. G., Krauss, D. A., & Burl, J. (2009). Training models in fo-rensic psychology. *Training and Education in Professional Psychology, 3*, 184–191. doi:10.1037/aDD14582

Fernandez, K., Davis, K. M., Conroy, M. A., & Boccaccini, M. T. (2009). A model for training graduate psychology students to become legally informed clinicians. *Journal of Forensic Psychology Practice, 9*, 57–69. doi:10.1080/15228930802427072.

Hedge, K. A., & Brodsky, S. L. (2013). Students at the elbow: Graduate student obser-vation of forensic assessments. *Professional Psychology: Research and Practice, 44*, 266–273.

Heilbrun, K., & Collins, S. (1995). Evaluations of trial competency and mental state at the time of the offense: Report characteristics. *Professional Psychology: Research and Practice, 26*, 61–67.

Heilbrun, K., Grisso, T., & Goldstein, A. (2009). *Foundations of forensic mental health assessment.* New York: Oxford.

Heilbrun, K., Kelley, S. M., Koller, J. P., Giallella, C., & Peterson, L. (2013). The role of university based forensic clinics. *International Journal of Law and Psychiatry, 36*, 195–200.

Melton, G. B., Petrila, J., Poythress, N. G., Slobogin, C., Otto, R. K., Mossman, D., & Condie, L. O. (2018). *Psychological evaluations for the courts: A handbook for mental health professionals and lawyers* (4th ed.). New York: Guilford.

Murrie, D. C., Boccaccini, M. T., Guarnera, L. A., & Rufino, K. A. (2013). Are forensic experts biased by the side that retained them? *Psychological Science, 24,* 1889–1897. doi:10.1177/0956797613481812

Otto, R. K., & Heilbrun, K. (2002). The practice of forensic psychology: A look toward the future in light of the past. *American Psychologist, 57,* 5–18. doi:10.1037//0003-066X.57.1.5

Packer, I. K. (2008). Specialized practice in forensic psychology: Opportunities and obstacles. *Professional Psychology: Research and Practice, 39,* 245–249. doi:10.1037/0735-7038

Texas Code of Criminal Procedure. (2019). Title 1, Chapter 46B, Incompetence to Stand Trial.

Texas Code of Criminal Procedure (2019). Title 1, Chapter 46C, Insanity Defense.

Texas Health & Safety Code. (1999). Section 571.003. https:https://codes.findlaw.com/tx/health-and-safety-code/health-safety-sect-571-003.html

5

Ohio's Criminal Justice Coordinating Center of Excellence

MARK R. MUNETZ, NATALIE BONFINE, RUTH H. SIMERA,
AND CHRISTOPHER NICASTRO* ■

Ohio has had a long history of collaborating with the state's universities, especially its six medical schools and their associated psychiatry residency programs. Toward the end of the twentieth century, the Ohio Department of Mental Health (ODMH; now the Ohio Department of Mental Health and Addiction Services [OMHAS]), led by Dr. Michael Hogan, had essentially completed the transition from a hospital-based to a community-based system of care. The role of the state hospitals had dramatically changed, with hospital closures and marked reductions in capacity. Given that Ohio is highly decentralized, with a system of single or multiple county mental health authorities (alcohol, drug addiction, and mental health services boards) that in many cases are predominantly funded by local taxes, the role of the state mental health authority was in question.

Leaders at the state were devising creative ways to guide and support the development of evidence-based and promising practices at the community level. Dr. Hogan recognized the important role of academic institutions as key partners in facilitating the statewide implementation of these practices. The state's approach to ensuring that communities had access to best practices in mental health and substance use treatment was to empower community–university partnerships called Coordinating Centers of Excellence (CCoEs). The CCoE effort was led at the state level by ODMH Medical Director, Dr. Dale Svendsen. Each CCoE focused around a various need or practice.

* The authors would like to thank Dr. Dale Svendsen for his vision and guidance in developing the Criminal Justice Coordinating Center of Excellence (CCoE). We are also grateful for the contributions of Dr. Michael Hogan in the preparation of materials for this chapter and for sharing his story on the origins of the Criminal Justice CCoE, which we have captured here.

In this chapter, we describe the development and evolution of the Ohio Criminal Justice CCoE. This Center was developed to promote jail diversion alternatives for people with serious mental illness and co-occurring disorders. We also discuss our current operations, our partners, and the impact of the Center, and we share some of the lessons we have learned over the past 19 years in operating the Center.

Coordinating Centers of Excellence

Using a theory of dissemination of innovation, the concept of CCoEs emerged. This theory of innovation suggested that the most effective strategy was to combine elements of unplanned or spontaneous diffusion along with more directed and managed dissemination (Rogers, 2003). The Department recognized that there were individuals and academic departments in both state and private universities with expertise, energy, and enthusiasm in disseminating particular evidence-based or promising practices. The idea was that the state would essentially empower those groups to serve as credible, flexible ambassadors of the state, convince others to take on the practice, and then help them to do so effectively.

The name that the ODMH came up with for these programs was carefully chosen. Describing oneself as excellent at a minimum is boastful and may appear arrogant, but it does not appear that the CCoEs were viewed negatively by Ohio's mental health community. The use of the word "Coordinating" may have been part of the reason. The CCoEs were not centers where patients came for excellent care. These centers instead helped the many community mental health agency partners they worked with to be or become excellent.

The Department began by seeking stakeholder input in the planning of the CCoEs. They identified several evidence-based and promising practice areas and charted them on a graph, with the degree of supporting evidence on the X axis and what they called "salience," meaning the perceived importance of the intervention, on the Y axis (see Figure 5.1). Integrated dual-diagnosis treatment for serious mental illness and co-occurring substance use disorder was an example of a practice that had substantial evidence and was highly salient. Jail diversion was listed as low on evidence and, perhaps surprisingly at least in retrospect, was rated on the low side in salience as well.

At the time the CCoEs were being created, one of us (Mark Munetz, MD) was Chief Clinical Officer for the Summit County Alcohol, Drug Addiction, and Mental Health Services (ADM) Board and Director of Community Psychiatry at Northeast Ohio Medical University (NEOMED). Dr. Munetz had played a lead role at the Board in helping the Akron Police Department implement the first "Memphis model" crisis intervention team (CIT) program in Ohio in May 2000. Along with his law enforcement partner, then Lt. Michael Woody from the Akron Police Department, Dr. Munetz began encouraging other counties to consider adopting the CIT model. At the same time, the Summit County ADM Board was working with Akron Municipal Court Judge Elinore Marsh Stormer to establish the first misdemeanor-level problem-solving mental health court in Ohio. Those

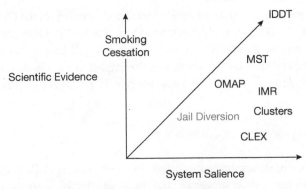

Figure 5.1 Ohio's Framework to Prioritizing EBP Promotion
Second Annual National Crisis Intervention Team (CIT) Conference, September 26, 2006

two programs seemed so promising that the ADM leadership approached ODMH and made a case for establishing a CCoE focused on jail diversion.

Unknown to those in Summit County, Dr. Hogan was in conversation with Dr. Hank Steadman, the founder of the National GAINS Center (now the Substance Abuse and Mental Health Services Administration [SAMHSA] GAINS Center). The GAINS Center is a federally funded organization that provides training and technical assistance across the country focused on addressing the needs of justice-involved individuals with serious mental illness and co-occurring substance use disorders. Director Hogan suggested to Dr. Steadman that a state-level CCoE focused on the intersection of mental health, co-occurring substance use, and criminal justice issues could be a state-level version of GAINS, what came to be called a "mini-GAINS Center." As such, in May 2001, the Summit County ADM Board was designated as the home of Ohio's Criminal Justice CCoE for Jail Diversion Alternatives, which almost immediately became known as the CJ CCoE. NEOMED was to operate the center. Funding from ODMH came from their federal block grant and was $200,000 a year.

The Sequential Intercept Model

Although both were considered promising and worth disseminating, neither CIT nor Mental Health Courts could be considered evidence-based practices in 2001, and, in fact, there is still some debate about their status today (Honegger, 2015; Watson, Compton, & Draine, 2017). Lacking a clear evidence-based practice, Dr. Hogan told Dr. Munetz, when announcing ODMH's decision to create the Center that, at a minimum, the CJ CCoE needed some sort of conceptual model to approach jail diversion. This demand was very much appreciated, as some ideas in that regard were already developing. Largely independent of the jail diversion initiatives, in 1999, the Summit County ADM Board had requested technical assistance from the GAINS Center on how to best address the justice-involved population with serious mental illness. The GAINS Center sent one of their senior consultants, Patricia Griffin, PhD, to provide what was then free consultation supported by SAMHSA funding. While the consultation was very helpful to the Summit County system and included encouragement to continue the planning then under way to start CIT and mental health court programs, the ongoing relationship between the Board and the GAINS Center, and between Drs. Munetz and Griffin in particular, turned out to be even more productive. From the consultation in Summit County and ongoing discussions between Drs. Munetz, Griffin, and, ultimately, Steadman came the *Sequential Intercept Model* (SIM), a simple framework on how to address a very complex problem (Munetz & Griffin, 2006).

In brief, the SIM details the progression of the criminal justice system, noting various points, or Intercepts, where the community mental health and substance use treatment system can coordinate with the criminal justice system to divert people in need to community-based treatment alternatives. In this model, the goal is diversion as early as possible to reduce inordinate involvement in the criminal justice system. An adequately supported community mental health and substance use treatment system serves as the Ultimate Intercept, now called "Intercept 0," where people in need and at risk of justice involvement may be identified and connected to appropriate community-based services (Abreu, Parker, Noether, Steadman, & Case, 2017; Bonfine, Wilson, & Munetz, in press).

The SIM has been used in a community action-planning workshop called Sequential Intercept Mapping. The SIM mapping workshop was developed by Policy Research Associates, Inc. (Griffin, Heilbrun, Mulvey, DeMatteo, & Schubert, 2015) and is now a core offering of the CJ CCoE. SIM mapping workshops promote dialogue and communication among stakeholders to address complex problems that affect justice and mental health systems (e.g., the overrepresentation of individuals with serious mental illness in the justice system). The primary objective is to minimize criminal justice involvement for persons with mental illness by enhancing collaboration across multiple systems and creating common visions and definitions for existing efforts from prearrest through reentry and community corrections. The day and a half workshop, which convenes a cross-section of key stakeholders, identifies challenges and opportunities and ultimately leads to the development of a Plan for Action. SIM mapping workshops strengthen local strategies to implement core services to address mental health, substance use, criminogenic, social, and environmental factors for justice-involved persons with mental illness and co-existing disorders.

Since its inception, the SIM has been widely used and adopted as an orienting framework for coordinating cross-systems responses to people with serious mental illness who are involved with the criminal justice system. The US Congress recently recognized the SIM and SIM mapping workshops as part of a comprehensive approach to community-based strategies to reduce justice involvement of

people with mental disorders (see Twenty-First Century Cures Act [2016] Public
Law 114-255, Title XIV, Subtitle B, §14021).

The Evolution of the Ohio Criminal Justice Coordinating
Center of Excellence

In 2001 when it was first funded, the CJ CCoE's initial role focused on helping
communities implement CIT programs in Ohio. Fortuitously, in June 2001,
a month after the CJ CCoE was launched, then Justice Evelyn Stratton of the
Supreme Court of Ohio began what came to be called the Advisory Committee
on Mental illness and the Courts (ACMIC) (Hawk, 2004). With endorsement
from the Chief Justice Thomas Moyer of the Supreme Court of Ohio and then
Governor Taft, ACMIC called together state leaders as well as representatives
from the county mental health and justice systems to improve services at the interface of the two systems. The CJ CCoE was a charter member of ACMIC. While
Justice Stratton supported the development of the Akron Mental Health Court,
she was not familiar with the CIT program before Dr. Munetz and Lt. Woody
shared the concepts and practice with her. She quickly became one of the biggest
advocates for CIT. Justice Stratton retired from the court in 2012, and the ACMIC
transitioned to become the Ohio Attorney General's Office Task Force on Criminal
Justice and Mental Illness. Retired Justice Stratton has remained the voice of the
Task Force, which is continuing under a new Attorney General in 2019.

Another important partnership emerged in the early development of the CJ
CCoE with the state chapter of the National Alliance on Mental Illness (NAMI).
NAMI Ohio learned about the CIT program and wanted to advocate across the
state to bring CIT to Ohio's many law enforcement agencies. With minimal debate, both the CJ CCoE and NAMI Ohio agreed they were stronger working together than in parallel and formed a partnership to promote and support CIT
development in the state. The CJ CCoE initially received funding through the
state mental health authority, and NAMI Ohio developed funding relationships
with the Ohio Attorney General and Office of Criminal Justice Services. Each
funder had somewhat different priorities. To maximize the impact of those funds
and the strengths of the CJ CCoE and NAMI Ohio, the CJ CCoE and NAMI
Ohio entered into subcontracts with each other, sending funds from the different
sources to one another. Braiding these diverse funding streams allowed both organizations to accomplish more together than either could alone.

NEOMED's role as an academic partner in operating the Center changed over
time as well. At first, much of the early work of the CJ CCoE happened in the community or in Akron at the ADM Board, an 18-mile drive from rural NEOMED.
Over time, however, NEOMED's role became increasingly important. Dr. Munetz
was appointed Chair of the Department of Psychiatry in 2007, and he spent
most of his time at NEOMED. The creation of a CJ CCoE website and the use of
NEOMED to house a growing resource library of books, videos, kits simulating
the voice hearing experience, and other materials has provided the Center's

partners important resources. The university helped create an Ohio CIT program video which proved valuable in the early dissemination of CIT. Being university-based has facilitated the Center getting additional external funding for programmatic and research efforts. The university's simulation center has helped develop role-play scenarios for local CIT programs. More recently, the CJ CCoE has been part of an intentional effort to partner with other programs in the Department of Psychiatry that have synergetic effects on each other. For example, the CJ CCoE helps police, jail, and court personnel be aware of coordinated specialty care programs for first-episode psychosis so that referrals can be made from the criminal justice system to these programs, which the Best Practices in Schizophrenia Treatment (BeST) Center has supported throughout Ohio.

Unexpectedly, as the CJ CCoE continued its evolution, the Department of Psychiatry at NEOMED became a significant partner with Peg's Foundation, previously known as The Margaret Clark Morgan Foundation. A local family foundation with a mission to improve mental health services in the northeast Ohio region, Peg's staff and board became increasingly interested in the criminal justice–mental health interface. With its mission to also have a national transformational impact, Peg's staff watched the work of the CJ CCoE and wanted to get involved. They developed relationships with state and national partners including now-retired Justice Stratton, the national and state Stepping Up Initiative, CIT International, and the Treatment Advocacy Center. As the primary funders of the Department of Psychiatry's BeST Center, Peg's Foundation has become a significant partner and helps now to fund a portion of the CJ CCoE. At this point our public–academic partnership is fully a public-private-academic partnership.

This may be ideal. Public mental health systems, private foundations, and universities like NEOMED have distinct but complementary missions. Typically, neither the state nor private funders want to provide ongoing infrastructure support for a center like the CJ CCoE. But such support is necessary if the Center is to offer most of its services at no cost to the local communities it serves, communities that are substantially underfunded. As natural as the partnership between the state agency and the university has been, there are state limitations based on its federal block grant funding and various administrative guidelines and university limitations in fitting a nonresearch, public service center within its structure. The benefits and challenges of the public–academic partnership are more thoroughly addressed later in this chapter. However, private philanthropy serves as a natural bridge between the two. Private foundation funding can be extremely flexible, allowing for creative use of funds. Private foundations can serve as advocates. Foundation and center staff have been able to partner in a process of discovery—looking for the best possible solutions for Ohio's communities by convening experts from other states, visiting sites in other states, and promoting significant dialogue among stakeholders. With a state and private funder, we have been able to have each say to the other "we will support this work if you do as well," making (once again) the whole greater than the sum of its parts.

Current Operations and Funding

As of July 2019, the Center has three full-time dedicated staff members: a Director, a Dissemination Coordinator, and a Research Coordinator. Dr. Munetz as Chair of the Department of Psychiatry provides oversight to the Center, and Department faculty are collaborators in evaluation and research efforts associated with the work of the center, including our mapping initiative. Our research partners have published in the academic literature and present research findings at local, state, national, and international meetings.

The Center also has an extensive, diverse roster of external consultants and facilitators who represent many disciplines and geographic locales around the state of Ohio, including retired Lt. Michael Woody who continues to serve as the statewide CIT Coordinator and law enforcement liaison. Additional consultants serve as facilitators of SIM mapping exercises, content experts, and providers of technical assistance to counties and jurisdictions all over the state on topics ranging from pretrial to reentry. Various community-based partners throughout the state contribute to the work of the Center as it has expanded well outside of Akron, Ohio.

The CJ CCoE has a Collaboration Board, which is a requirement of projects funded by Edward Byrne Memorial Justice Assistance Grants (Byrne JAG) through the Ohio Office of Criminal Justice Services. The CJ CCoE found great benefit in convening quarterly meetings among our collaborators, including local (Wood County Alcohol, Drug Addiction, and Mental Health Services Board and consumers), regional (Peg's Foundation), state (Ohio Department of Rehabilitation and Correction, Ohio Department of Mental Health and Addiction Services [OMHAS], Office of Criminal Justice Services, NAMI Ohio, and Ohio Stepping Up Initiative), and national (Treatment Advocacy Center) representatives and content experts (SIM mapping facilitators and technical assistance consultants) and has maintained this Board regardless of current Byrne JAG funding. These meetings provide an excellent opportunity to hear from community partners that have participated in SIM mapping, gain input on planning and program improvements, and maintain up-to-date cross-systems information at the state level.

The OMHAS has continued annual funding to the Center, now at $190,000 per year, 100% of which passes through the Summit County ADM Board through a subcontract agreement. A $10,000 annual reduction (from $200,000 to $190,000) occurred through OMHAS in Fiscal Year 2009 and has since remained stable. OMHAS assigns a liaison to the Center, often referred to as a "lead," who approves the funding applications and serves as a central point of contact for Center staff. The lead also participates on the Center's Collaboration Board and is readily accessible when guidance is needed. The Center provides semi-annual reports to OMHAS as part of the terms of funding but also distributes a variety of self-generated reports to state agency representatives and community stakeholders to highlight the work of the Center and the trends and priorities emerging across the state. These reports have been used by state entities to aid in federal funding applications and to encourage state funding for systems-level needs.

Through a 5-year award to the NEOMED Department of Psychiatry, Peg's Foundation earmarked $150,000 per year for the CJ CCoE through June 2023 ($750,000 total). Peg's investment in the CJ CCoE is more akin to OMHAS's current investment in the CJ CCoE than it is to a grant, as it is aimed at supporting the broader work of the Center and enhancing the Center's capacity while ensuring it has a funding foundation to consistently maintain operations. All other support to the Center is and has been through grants, such as the Edward Byrne Memorial Justice Assistance Grants (Byrne JAG) through the Office of Criminal Justice Services (OCJS) for SIM mapping, and Justice Mental Health Collaboration Program (JMHCP) awards through the Bureau of Justice Assistance for expansion of the CJ CCoE to evaluate Sequential Intercept Mapping, enhance technical assistance activities, and target county-level work on jail data collection and cross-systems information sharing. The JMHCP awards have been through partnership applications with OCJS (the applicant), OMHAS (the mental health partner), and the CJ CCoE (the implementing agency).

The Impact of the CJ CCoE

The services provided and the impact to Ohio through the CJ CCoE and its partners are far-reaching. Starting with CIT, Ohio has trained nearly 13,000 sworn law enforcement officers since the first class in Akron in May 2000. Today all 88 Ohio counties have trained CIT officers. CIT is largely organized by local alcohol, drug addiction, and mental health services board areas, of which there are 50 in Ohio. Of those, 45 provide CIT training and designate a county or multicounty CIT program coordinator, as well as coordinators in many law enforcement jurisdictions. CIT Program Coordinators submit completed training rosters to the CJ CCoE and the law enforcement liaison, who compiles and reports aggregate training data quarterly. Included in these reports are the rosters of law enforcement agencies participating in CIT and the percentage of law enforcement jurisdictions within each county that are participating in CIT. For the counties or board areas that do not sponsor their own training, officers are able to receive training in neighboring counties, still at no cost to them. The CJ CCoE and NAMI Ohio collaborate through state grants to make available mini-grants to help defray costs of CIT training and to offer an annual statewide CIT Advanced Training Conference.

The CJ CCoE and NAMI Ohio coordinate semi-annual statewide meetings of CIT Coordinators, a gathering of law enforcement, mental health, probation/parole, corrections, advocacy coordinators, and occasionally other stakeholders from around the state to discuss topics of interest or impact to CIT. With direction and leadership from the CJ CCoE, the CIT Coordinators group has been a keystone to the bottom-up energy of CIT in Ohio, drafting an early consensus document on the key elements of CIT which predated the national CIT Core Elements (Dupont et al., 2007) and designing a CIT Peer Review process, Ohio's version of continuous quality improvement for CIT. The Peer Review process, initiated in 2010, includes (1) a self-assessment, typically completed by the CIT Program

Coordinator and local steering committee; (2) a desk audit of all CIT training and programmatic materials completed by the statewide consultant/CIT Coordinator and two experienced CIT peers, typically one representing law enforcement and one mental health; (3) an observation of the local CIT training (if possible); and (4) a site visit, including the reviewers and local steering committee, to review the drafted report which summarizes the strengths and areas for improvement for the program. Twenty-one board-area programs covering 32 of Ohio's 88 counties have participated in Peer Reviews. Beyond these formal products and often upon request from the CJ CCoE, Ohio CIT coordinators give their time throughout the state to other county programs by mentoring new coordinators and new CIT programs, participating as instructors in the CJ CCoE-sponsored CIT Coordinator Course and CIT Dispatch Training of Trainers Course, and providing technical assistance to one another in areas of program development.

The Center began offering an 8-hour CIT Coordinators Course in 2017, and it has provided this training four times, with 105 individuals completing the training across 34 of the board areas and the Ohio Department of Rehabilitation and Correction. Similarly, the Center began offering an 8-hour CIT Dispatch Training of Trainers in 2017, and it has provided this training three times, with 76 individuals completing it across 28 board areas. Additional activities associated with CIT dissemination include the lending library, hearing distressing voices simulation kits, a robust website (www.neomed.edu/cjccoe/) with training and technical assistance resources, mentoring, CIT Coordinators semi-annual meeting, quarterly newsletter, email distribution list, and technical assistance. Technical assistance is available from the Center through staff or consultant time, website resources, training, email distribution, video and telephone conferencing, the lending library, and other forms of resource distribution (e.g., publications, books, videos, etc.). The CIT Coordinator, who has the greatest flexibility among the consultants, submits monthly reports of activities to the Center along with monthly invoices. Other independent consultants operate on an hourly fee-for-service basis and submit agreed-upon products or reports associated with each activity. Members of the CIT Coordinators group provide volunteer technical assistance and peer assistance to other communities.

CJ CCoE staff and 12 external consultants cooperate to facilitate systems mapping exercises. Consultants are a vital piece of this work, bringing depth and breadth of content expertise in areas of pretrial functions, prosecution, forensic psychology, prevention and training, law enforcement, substance use treatment, defense law, mental health treatment and administration, and more. The CJ CCoE has completed 41 systems mapping exercises across 33 counties. Most of the mappings (28) have targeted the adult mental health and justice system collaborations. However, the CJ CCoE adapted the mapping workshop exercise to meet a pressing need associated with the opiate epidemic (Bonfine, Munetz, & Simera, 2018). After receiving financial support from state partners to complete a pilot opioid-focused SIM in one county, the Center has now completed 11 mapping exercises to address the opioid crisis and related substance use problems at the interface of the criminal justice system. The Center also adapted the model for the juvenile mental health and justice systems and has completed two such exercises. Evaluations of Ohio's systems mapping workshops are under way, but initial findings suggest that the exercise is well-received by participants, and it has reportedly improved collaborative efforts and enhanced community programming and practices to address the needs of the target population (Bonfine & Nadler, 2019).

The extensive SIM mapping completed by the CJ CCoE has prompted its significant involvement in a number of important initiatives. Ohio, in part based on strong support from Peg's Foundation, has become an active state in the Stepping Up Initiative. The CJ CCoE director serves on the Stepping Up Ohio Steering Committee. Based on key gaps and priorities identified in multiple counties, the CJ CCoE has engaged in work with its funders to address the Crisis Response System in Ohio; the Center is also actively working with the Treatment Advocacy Center to promote and implement Assisted Outpatient Treatment (AOT) throughout Ohio following a change in the state's civil commitment law. AOT is seen as both a way to prevent justice involvement altogether and prevent recidivism upon reentry (Gilbert et al., 2010; Swartz et al., 2001). Recognizing that Ohio, like most states, is using a significant portion of its limited state hospital beds for competency restoration of individuals charged with a misdemeanor (Gowensmith, Frost, Speelman, & Therson, 2016), the CJ CCoE has participated in the state's examination of alternative ways to address this issue in hopes of making hospital beds more accessible to civil patients. The lack of continuity of pharmacotherapy for individuals confined to local jails has also been identified as a significant issue in Ohio, particularly access to clozapine and long-acting injectible antipsychotic medications. The Center is working with state and local partners to address this issue and, with its partners at Peg's Foundation, has engaged in advocacy to eliminate the Medicaid Inmate Exclusion (Munetz, Messamore, & Dugan, 2018).

Why a Public Behavioral Health–University Partnership?

Basing statewide training and technical assistance centers at a university has advantages. A university brings instant credibility and, to some extent, prestige to such an enterprise. More importantly, a university's tripartite mission of education, research, and service aligns closely with the mission of the state mental health and addiction authority and matches and enhances the work of a training and technical assistance center. Furthermore, an unanticipated benefit of placing the CCoEs within Ohio medical schools' departments of psychiatry has been the increased emphasis within these departments on community-based psychiatry and the importance of addressing serious mental illness within community settings. Current chairs of departments of psychiatry at Ohio's six allopathic medical schools include three who helped establish CCoEs—including the Criminal Justice CCoE at NEOMED (Dr. Mark Munetz), the Center for Evidence-Based Practices at Case Western Reserve University (Dr. Robert Ronis), and the Mental Illness/Intellectual Disabilities Coordinating Center of Excellence at Wright

State (Dr. Julie Gentile). These chairs include in their mission recruiting medical students to psychiatry and residents to work in the public sector.

While the CJ CCoE and centers like it largely focus on the current, existing workforce, its placement in a university also offers opportunities to begin training the emerging workforce. Teaching resources including academic information technology at NEOMED have enhanced the work of our Center. One example was the creation of an Ohio CIT video, which has been helpful in CIT dissemination in our state. The video script was written by CJ CCoE staff but filmed and edited by academic technology staff who subsequently updated some of the captions. Access to the interuniversity library is another important resource for the CJ CCoE, as we have access to scientific literature not easily accessed by either community mental health or justice system personnel. We share that literature as part of our resource library.

While the CJ CCoE was established to disseminate jail diversion programs across the state, even two decades later the evidence base for the effectiveness of such programs is limited. Placing the Center at a university has facilitated partnership with research faculty interested in the work of the Center. The conceptual model guiding the work of the Center, the SIM, was published in a prominent psychiatry journal, widely disseminated, and led our partners/mentors at the SAMHSA GAINS Center and Policy Research Associates, Inc. to operationalize it as a mapping workshop. Only in the past several years have researchers in the Department begun to do systematic research on the effectiveness of mapping. NEOMED faculty have also been significant contributors to the emerging scientific literature studying the impact of CIT programs, mental health courts, issues around criminogenic risk, and AOT. If the training and Technical Assistance Center were not embedded within a university, this research partnership would probably have not been as successful.

Core funding for the CJ CCoE typically comes from the state mental health authority using federal block grant dollars, although it has been supported using state general revenue funds at times. The initial funding began almost 20 years ago. It was never increased and, after a 5% reduction, has remained flat year after year. Even with the modest inflation in this current era, costs go up considerably over time—so training and technical assistance centers must seek additional funds to remain viable and grow. The CJ CCoE has been successful in doing that, but it has not been easy. The success is the result of developing strong credibility over many years such that state agencies see the Center's value. This is accompanied by developing strong relationships with many partner organizations. Universities also have lobbyists (i.e., government relations officers) who can help build relationships not only with the executive departments of state government but also with legislators. In a term-limited state legislature, as we have in Ohio, it is not uncommon for a state representative or senator to find his or her way into a cabinet position in subsequent years. Relationship building through the university's government relations officer can help a great deal in maintaining program funding.

We have learned that another advantage of the public–university collaboration is the ability to seek external funds. Over the life of the CJ CCoE, some grants that the Center was able to obtain required that they be based at a university; others required a unit of government to apply. The US Bureau of Justice Assistance Justice and Mental Health Collaboration Program grants is a prime example of the latter. The CJ CCoE has successfully written such grant applications, which were then submitted through a collaboration with two of our funders (at the state mental health authority as well as the Ohio Office of Criminal Justice Services). Seeking grant opportunities within a university is not without challenges. There is the expectation in universities that government grants are accompanied by substantial reimbursement of administrative overhead and facility support, so-called indirect costs. While indirect support for basic research is a negotiated rate with federal agencies that helps support the significant infrastructure of a research university, the state and federal agencies supporting the CJ CCoE do not support administrative overhead at the same level as research grants. Senior leaders at the university did not always appreciate the difference between research and the community service the CJ CCoE was providing. It has been a continuing challenge on how best to inform university leaders of the nature of the work and convince them that the service provided by the Center was congruent with the university's mission. Enlisting the university's government affairs office has helped in communicating the importance of the work of the Center.

Naïvely, we tried for many years to get partners at the state to similarly collaborate to fund our effort. Conceptually, we wondered why state agencies such as the state Department of Mental Health, and the state Department of Addiction Services and Public Safety (the home of the Office of Criminal Justice Services) couldn't pool resources and collectively fund the work of the CJ CCoE. The possibility of "blended" funding—putting funds from multiple state agencies in a single pot—has never come to pass. It simply is not how state government works, at least in Ohio. Each state grant has its own specific set of deliverables, and tracking and accounting for blended funds is not practical. Instead, a smarter approach, and one that has served us well, turned out to be getting core annual support through block grant dollars from mental health, repeated success receiving competitive grants from the state criminal justice services agency, and also using federal funds through the Edward Byrne Memorial Justice Assistance Grants. In addition, we have had some success getting direct funding from the Ohio Attorney General's office, but more often such funds are obtained by NAMI Ohio and passed through to the CJ CCoE. So, while state government seems unable, in part because of limitations from federal funders, to "blend" funding together to support the Center, with hard work on our part we have been able to "braid" funds from multiple funders, each grant with its own set of deliverables, to expand the scope of work of the Center (for more discussion of blended and braided funding, see https://workforce.urban.org/strategy/blended-and-braided-funding). We did have some success in shared funding when two state agencies agreed to partner on our behalf for the Bureau of Justice Assistance Justice and Mental Health Collaboration grants noted earlier. Those agencies, particularly through the lead contacts we have at the two state agencies, were eager to support our application and have been active participants in the projects supported by the federal grants.

Challenges and Lessons Learned

We have encountered several hard challenges over the two decades of operating the CJ CCoE. The first was the recognition that few, if any, funders want to maintain a base infrastructure of a center like the CJ CCoE. The beauty of a state-supported but university-operated training and technical assistance center is that we could offer needed expertise, support, and resources to underfunded communities at no monetary charge to the communities. State leaders, to varying degrees, had an expectation that communities should or would pay for such services. This may appear to be a philosophical debate, but in reality if the CJ CCoE's funding was dependent on convincing counties to pay us for our services, it would likely (1) not have sustained the Center, (2) have diverted our attention from our core mission as we chased contracts, and (3) have diverted dollars that the counties desperately needed to support their services. So, while we were as entrepreneurial as possible in pursuing grants and grant funds received by our county partners, we mostly thrived by offering our services for "free." However, these free services were only offered to committed communities that were willing to put in the effort to do the hard work of collaboration and program development.

The second challenge has been that state administrations change, and with such change come new people, new philosophies, and the need to reassert the added value that the CJ CCoE offered the state and its counties. Since the inception of the CJ CCoE, Ohio has had four governors and four directors of the state mental health authority. Different state directors had different levels of enthusiasm for the academic partnerships. There appears to be a tendency over time in state government for state officials to want to bring responsibility back to central government and delegate less to academic partners. This may reflect a naturally swinging pendulum. At times this tendency has led to frustration that the experienced leaders and consultants of the CJ CCoE are typically not consulted when state agencies make decisions. This tendency has been countered, in our case, by the continued presence of a retired Supreme Court of Ohio justice and a director of the state NAMI affiliate who have partnered with our Center through all these administrations and have consistently supported our work. Most recently, this has been manifested by the appointment of the CJ CCoE Director to the Steering Committee and Core Team of Ohio's Stepping Up Initiative. Stepping Up in Ohio is the most visible initiative being driven by multiple state cabinet-level officials along with leaders in community mental health and criminal justice.

The third and perhaps hardest problem is that after nearly two decades of work, the problem of the overrepresentation of people with mental illness in the criminal justice system persists. As much as we have worked to address this problem, there are still jails and prisons with too many people with serious mental illness. The challenge for our Center is to show the positive impact of the programs we promote. Research suggests, for example, that CIT programs may not substantially reduce arrest rates of people with severe mental illness, but they may decrease the rare officer-involved shooting and more common uses of force, may decrease use of SWAT, and perhaps most importantly may increase connecting people with severe mental illness to treatment rather than taking no action and saying the situation was resolved (Arey, Wilder, Normore, Iannazzo, & Javidi, 2015; Canada, Angell, & Watson, 2010, 2011; Compton et al., 2011, 2014; Morabito et al., 2012; Teller, Munetz, Gil, & Ritter, 2006; Watson et al., 2010). However, this wicked problem will not be completely solved until some of the big societal problems associated with serious mental illness are addressed (e.g., poverty, homelessness, recurrent trauma, and victimization).

We have learned many lessons over the years. These are detailed in the following sections.

Fostering Partnerships at Multiple Levels Is Essential

Finding a Supreme Court justice who embraced the issue of reducing justice involvement of people with mental illness was incredibly lucky. While every state may not have such a champion, the growing Psychiatrists Judges Leadership Initiative supported by the Council of State Government's Justice Center and the American Psychiatric Association Foundation has been identifying and educating interested judges throughout the country. Anyone working on this issue should try to find a judge to help lead and promote jail diversion efforts. Judges in particular have convening power; when they invite various stakeholders to meetings, even very important public officials tend to show up. Even one influential champion is tremendously helpful. Having more than one champion representing different stakeholder groups is even more helpful. We were both fortunate and smart to collaborate with a strong state NAMI chapter whose advocacy and influence was invaluable. We were also fortunate to have a nationally renowned consumer advocate, Dr. Fred Frese, speak on our behalf regularly wherever he went. Having family and consumer voices advocating for the work we were supporting was essential. While few states may have a Justice Stratton or a consumer voice like the late Dr. Frese, many states may find a police chief, sheriff, or jail administrator, or there may be a public defender, county prosecutor, or state representative whose voice is heard who can help champion the issue.

When the national Stepping Up initiative began, Justice Stratton used her influence with state leaders for Ohio to encourage its counties to participate. Forming a state-level Stepping Up Steering Committee, retired Justice Stratton enlisted full support from the state director of mental health, the attorney general, and multiple other state directors. In the background, funding for this effort was from Peg's Foundation. Arguably, Peg's Foundation was primed to support Stepping Up because of their relationship with the medical school and the work of the CJ CCoE. One relationship leads to the next. One never knows exactly where these relationships will lead, but for us, it has led to more opportunities.

While formal agreements are necessary for funds to move between organizations, much of our work has been through informal partnerships and by building a network of local community stakeholders. Soon after the founding of the Center, together with NAMI Ohio we began hosting CIT Coordinator meetings. We have never rigidly defined who is a CIT Coordinator, wanting to grow the role in law enforcement, mental health, and advocacy. The biannual meetings of this grassroots learning community have been well-attended, and we believe this has helped Ohio evolve effective CIT programs around the state.

One of the most important keys to our success echoes a famous Woody Allen quote, that "80% of success is showing up." Traveling frequently to our state capital for state-level meetings was important. More important was taking opportunities to demonstrate our collective expertise so we were seen as an essential voice at the table. A corollary was making ourselves available at the local county level. From the beginning of the CJ CCoE, one or more of us traveled regularly to share our expertise and passion with local communities. Most effective was going in pairs. This varied from the early travels of Dr. Munetz and Lt. Woody, where they could model the partnership between police and mental health and have credibility with both stakeholder groups. Even more powerful was when one of us, most recently Director Ruth Simera, could attend county meetings with state leaders like Justice Stratton as part of the Stepping Up initiative.

While maintaining relationships with top state officials was important, having real working relationships with the staff at the state agencies with whom we worked most closely was even more important. These staff, with whom we were generally able to view issues and solutions in a similar way, have been great advocates with their leaders who control the purse strings. A key example is our primary contact at our lead funder, OMHAS. The CJ CCoE has had four OMHAS leads since the inception of the Center, three who served for extended periods of time, including our current lead and co-author on this chapter, Christopher Nicastro. The OMHAS lead has served as a boundary spanner between the state bureaucracy and the work of the CJ CCoE. Over time, with each, trust has been established and the lead has served as translator, explainer, and advocate for all parties. This close working relationship has helped our Center have the vision and flexibility needed to respond to emergent issues. For instance, we coordinated training for public defenders on mental illness and the mental health system when we learned of a need. Also, as the opioid crisis emerged in Ohio, we were poised to implement our mapping workshops with communities to address the needs of people at risk for opioid use disorder or overdose.

KNOW AND COMMUNICATE THE VALUE THAT YOU BRING

The CJ CCoE found itself somewhat stuck during the interval of the Great Recession between 2008 and 2012. Having helped develop the SIM, the CJ CCoE wanted to move into conducting mapping workshops in Ohio, as was happening in several other states, including our neighbors in Pennsylvania. However, state mental health leaders were concerned that mapping workshops would lead to counties identifying large unmet needs that would require funding. Such funding was not available at that time. The Center leadership failed to convince state leaders that times of limited resources were actually ideal times to conduct mapping exercises because such exercises identify gaps in almost all communities, including relatively "quick fixes," necessary changes in policy or procedures, or redistribution of existing personnel or funds that do not require new dollars. The CJ CCoE failed to explain the value of community collaboration stimulated by mapping exercises that would have been particularly useful in times of resource scarcity.

CREATE A COMMUNITY OF EXPERTS

As we initiated our efforts to disseminate CIT statewide and later, as we did Mapping workshops and provided technical assistance as communities worked on implementing their action plans, we used a two-step process to facilitate and accelerate the work. Step one was to take advantage of a small but growing group of content experts in a specific intervention or focus area. We began with our law enforcement liaison and experts in specialty dockets through the Supreme Court of Ohio. When we received training in mapping from the Policy Research Associates, Inc., we chose an interprofessional group of facilitators representing mental health (including forensic mental health), law enforcement, prosecutor, and pretrial services, as well as defense counsel, substance use treatment, and probation and parole. We identified privacy as a major issue impacting information sharing, so we added a mental health attorney to our cadre of experts able to offer technical assistance.

In addition to these experts we could deploy to provide technical assistance to communities requesting help, we identified knowledgeable people in these different areas and others (e.g., jail administrators, emergency service directors, and, with the emerging opioid epidemic, experts in substance use disorders). These regional experts were generally willing to volunteer to share their experience and expertise with peers in neighboring communities. With the advent of videoconferencing, we have recently begun using regional experts on a particular issue to provide web-based technical assistance to one or two targeted counties looking to solve a similar problem or develop a similar program. Recent examples of successful video technical assistance efforts include consultation on validated screening at jail booking or co-responder teams pairing police with mental health crisis workers.

Finally, we have learned, and we teach when we do mapping workshops, that the key to success in diversion efforts is for everyone, from every stakeholder group (mental health, substance use, criminal justice, individuals with mental disorders and their family members) to do their work differently. We have assembled staff, consultants, and collaborating organizations to reflect this diverse group of people coming together. Our current Collaboration Board includes representatives from psychiatry, social work, social science research, law enforcement, pretrial services; a prosecuting attorney (who was a former public defender); representatives from correctional mental health; an individual in recovery from a co-occurring disorder; and a family advocate. However, not everyone is adept at working across systems. Finding the right staff and consultants who could be comfortable with and effective in talking with mental health professionals, police officers, judges, and family advocates was not always easily accomplished. And it is essential that the staff and partners are dedicated to addressing the issue, even if that means doing things in a different way. Fortunately, for most of its first two decades of operation, this has been a rare problem.

CONCLUSION

For almost two decades Ohio's CJ CCoE has provided resources, expertise, and technical assistance to counties attempting to address the overrepresentation of people with serious mental illness and co-occurring substance use disorders in the criminal justice system. The vision and leadership of Drs. Hogan, Svendsen, and Steadman to develop a state-level training and technical assistance center to complement the work of a national center like the SAMHSA GAINS Center has been realized to a large extent. As the recent report of SAMHSA's Interdepartmental Serious Mental Illness Coordinating Committee (2017) suggests, state mental health and substance use directors should consider using federal block grant dollars to support such centers.

State-level centers appear to be at the right scale to be maximally effective. Even in a state like Ohio, with a strong tradition of local control at the county level, within the state everyone is operating under the same laws. Law enforcement training, courts (to some degree), the bar, and other licensing authorities are all at a state level. Larger regional/multistate centers may provide effective training, useful resources, and publications addressing issues common to many states, and technical assistance to Centers such as the CJ CCoE, but ongoing support of local program implementation, which often hinges on relationships and timely access to resources and technical assistance, seems most efficient at the state level.

Finally, we have found that being a statewide training and technical assistance Center at a university is ideal. The NEOMED Department of Psychiatry's focus on community-based psychiatry, our service-oriented mission, and dedication to aiding communities aligns with the mission of our state partners. We have also been able to make use of academic resources, grant and funding opportunities and other partnerships, including with a local private foundation. The confluence of these partnerships, built over time and maintained with care, have helped our Center thrive.

REFERENCES

Abreu, D., Parker, T. W., Noether, C. D., Steadman, H. J., & Case, B. A. (2017). Revising the paradigm for jail diversion for people with mental and substance use disorders: Intercept 0. *Behavioral Sciences and the Law, 35*, 380–395. doi:https://doi.org/10.1002/bsl.2300

Arey, J. B., Wilder, A. H., Normore, A. H., Iannazzo, M. D., & Javidi, M. (2015). Crisis Intervention Teams: An evolution of leadership in community policing. *Policing: A Journal of Policy and Practice, 10*(2), 143–149. doi:10.1093/police/pav037

Bonfine, N., Munetz, M. R., & Simera, R. H. (2018). Sequential intercept mapping: Developing systems level solutions for the opioid epidemic. *Psychiatric Services, 69*, 1124–1126.

Bonfine, N., & Nadler, N. (2019). The perceived impact of sequential intercept mapping on communities collaborating to address adults with mental illness in the criminal justice system. *Administration and Policy in Mental Health and Mental Health Services Research, 46*(5), 569–579.

Bonfine, N., Wilson, A. B., Munetz, M. R. (2020). Meeting the needs of Justice-Involved People With Serious Mental Illness Within Community Behavioral Health Systems. *Psychiatric Services, 71*, 355–363.

Canada, K. E., Angell, B., & Watson, A. C. (2010). Crisis intervention teams in Chicago: Successes on the ground. *Journal of Police Crisis Negotiations, 10*, 86–100.

Canada, K. E., Angell, B., & Watson, A. C. (2011). Intervening at the entry point: Differences in how CIT trained and non-CIT trained officers describe responding to mental health-related calls. *Community Mental Health Journal, 48*(6), 746–755.

Compton, M. T., Bakeman, R., Broussard, B., Hankerson-Dyson, D., Husbands, L., Krishan, S., . . . Watson, A. C. (2014). The police-based Crisis Intervention Team (CIT) model: II. Effects on level of force and resolution, referral and arrest. *Psychiatric Services, 65*(4), 523–529.

Compton, M. T., Demir Neubert, B. N., Broussard, B., McGriff, J. A., Morgan, R., & Oliva, J. R. (2011). Use of force preferences and perceived effectiveness of actions among Crisis Intervention Team (CIT) police officers and non-CIT officers in an escalating psychiatric crisis involving a subject with schizophrenia. *Schizophrenia Bulletin, 37*(4), 737–745.

Dupont, R., Cochran, S., Pillsbury, S., Munetz, M. R., Woody, M., Lott-Haynes, N., . . . Forsyth-Stephens, A. (2007). *Crisis Intervention Team core elements*. Memphis, TN: University of Memphis. http://www.citinternational.org/Memphis-Model-Core-Elements

Gowensmith, W. N., Frost, L. E., Speelman, D. W., & Therson, D. E. (2016). Lookin' for beds in all the wrong places: Outpatient competency restoration as a promising approach to modern challenges. *Psychology, Public Policy, and Law, 22*(3), 293–305.

Gilbert, A. R., Moser, L. L., Van Dorn, R. A., Swanson, J. W., Wilder, C. M., Clark Robbins, P., . . . Swartz, M.S. (2010). Reductions in arrest under assisted outpatient treatment in New York. *Psychiatric Services, 61*(10), 996–999.

Griffin, P. A., Heilbrun, K., Mulvey, E. P., DeMatteo, D., & Schubert, C. A. (2015). *The Sequential Intercept Model and criminal justice: Promoting community alternatives for individuals with serious mental illness.* New York: Oxford University Press.

Hawk, K. L. (2004). The Supreme Court of Ohio Advisory Committee on Mentally Ill in the Courts: A catalyst for change. *Capital University Law Review, 32*, 1079–1083.

Honegger, L. N. (2015). Does the evidence support the case for mental health courts? A review of the literature. *Law and Human Behavior, 39*(5), 478–488.

Interdepartmental Serious Mental Illness Coordinating Committee. (2017). *The way forward: Federal action for a system that works for all people living with SMI and SED and their families and caregivers.* Rockville, MD: Substance Abuse and Mental Health Services Administration. https://www.samhsa.gov/ismicc

Morabito, M. S., Kerr, A. N., Watson, A., Draine, J., Ottati, V., & Angell, B. (2012). Crisis Intervention Teams and people with mental illness: Exploring the factors that influence the use of force. *Crime & Delinquency, 58*(1), 57–77.

Munetz, M. R., & Griffin, P. A. (2006). Use of the sequential intercept model as an approach to decriminalization of people with serious mental illness. *Psychiatric Services, 57*(4), 544–549. doi:10.1176/ps.2006.57.4.544

Munetz, M. R., Messamore, E., & Dugan, S. E. (2018). *Bringing treatment parity to jail inmates with schizophrenia*. Philadelphia: Scattergood Foundation. https://www.scattergoodfoundation.org/publication/bringing-treatment-parity-to-jail-inmates-with-schizophrenia/

Rogers, E. M. (2003). *Diffusion of innovations* (5th ed.). New York: Free Press.

Swartz, M. S., Swanson, J. W., Hiday, V. A., Wagner, H. R., Burns, B. J., & Borum, R. (2001). A randomized controlled trial of outpatient commitment in North Carolina. *Psychiatric Services, 52*(3), 325–329.

Teller, J. L. S., Munetz, M. R., Gil, K. M., & Ritter, C. (2006). Crisis intervention team training for police officers responding to mental disturbance calls. *Psychiatric Services, 57*(2), 232–237.

Twenty-First Century Cures Act of 2016, Pub. L. No. 114-255, Subtitle B, § 14021 (2016).

Watson, A. C., Compton, M. T., & Draine, J. N. (2017). The crisis intervention team (CIT) model: An evidence-based policing practice? *Behavioral Sciences and the Law, 35*, 431–441.

Watson, A. C., Ottati, V. C., Morabito, M., Draine, J., Kerr, A. N., & Angell, B. (2010). Outcomes of police contacts with persons with mental illness: The impact of CIT. *Administration and Policy in Mental Health and Mental Health Services Research, 37*(4), 302–317.

6

University of California Davis Forensic Psychiatry and California Department of State Hospitals Collaboration

Achieving Mutual Respect and Harmony

CHARLES SCOTT, BARBARA MCDERMOTT, AND KATHERINE WARBURTON ■

PURPOSE OF THE COLLABORATION

The purpose of the collaboration between the University of California, Davis, Medical Center (UCDMC Davis) and the California Department of State Hospitals (DSH) is to research, identify, and implement effective approaches for the assessment, management, and treatment of individuals in California's long-term psychiatric facilities. These goals are in concert with the California DSH mission statement: "To provide evaluation and treatment in a safe and responsible manner, by leading innovation and excellence across a continuum of care and settings" (California Department of State Hospitals, 2019). A more detailed description of both agencies will assist the reader in better understanding the origins and evolution of this collaboration.

The UCDMC Davis Medical Center

UCDMC is an academic medical center located in Sacramento, California, that provides specialty care in 150 fields. The UCDMC Department of Psychiatry and

Behavioral Sciences provides residency training in multiple areas of psychiatry, including a 1-year accredited fellowship in forensic psychiatry. The forensic psychiatry division and fellowship training program was founded in 1996, under the leadership of Richard Yarvis, MD. Dr. Yarvis, a board-certified adult psychiatrist with added qualifications in forensic psychiatry, has published extensively on issues related to forensic offenders and has developed important ties to leaders and administrators responsible for providing care to individuals involved in the criminal justice system throughout Northern California.

In 1998, Charles Scott, MD, was recruited as the UCDMC forensic psychiatry fellowship director. National accreditation from the American Council on Graduate Medical Education (ACGME) was obtained that same year. ACGME has core program requirements for accreditation that include providing forensic psychiatry fellows exposure to individuals involved in the criminal justice system. The Sacramento County Jail and Napa State Hospital (NSH) were both selected as training sites to meet this requirement.

In 2001, Barbara McDermott, PhD, was recruited as a full-time faculty member to serve as forensic psychiatry research director within the UC Davis forensic psychiatry division. Dr. McDermott was initially assigned to conduct research at NSH. The evolution of her role is detailed later.

The Department of State Hospitals

The DSH manages the California state hospital system, which provides mental health services to patients admitted into DSH facilities. Originally designated as the Department of Mental Health (DMH), the system reorganized in 2012. Currently, DSH oversees five state hospitals: Atascadero State Hospital (ASH), Coalinga State Hospital (CSH), Metropolitan State Hospital (MSH; so called because it is located in metropolitan Los Angeles), NSH, and Patton State Hospital (PSH), each named for the location of the hospital. With the reorganization to an "enterprise system" (DSH; an effort to organize all hospitals to adopt comparable policies and procedures), names of the hospitals were altered slightly, although they all maintained the name of their location. As of 2018, DSH employed more than 11,000 staff and served more than 12,000 patients annually in a 24/7 hospital system.

Patients admitted to DSH are involuntarily committed for treatment by a criminal or civil court judge. More than 90% of DSH patients are under a forensic commitment, meaning that the criminal court system has mandated that they be psychiatrically hospitalized. Forensic commitment categories include individuals found incompetent to stand trial (IST), not guilty by reason of insanity (NGRI), and mentally disordered offender (MDO) (a civil commitment for offenders paroled to the mental health system because of dangerousness due to their severe mental illness). In addition to these forensic commitments, DSH treats patients who have been classified by a judge or jury as sexually violent predators (SVPs); this treatment is provided in one facility designed and built specifically for this purpose. These patients have completed their prison sentences for committing crimes enumerated under the Sexually Violent Predator Act and are committed to DSH for treatment until a judge deems they are no longer a threat to the community. Other forensic commitments include patients referred from the state prison system for treatment, and patients not able to be restored to competence but too dangerous to be released into the community.

The remainder of the department's population has been psychiatrically committed in civil court for having a mental disorder that results in their being a danger to themselves or others or gravely disabled. These patients are commonly referred to as having Lanterman-Petris-Short (LPS) commitments.

WHEN AND WHY THE COLLABORATION BEGAN

The original collaboration, between the UC Davis forensic psychiatry division and NSH began in 1998. NSH was opened on November 15, 1875, as a 500-bed psychiatric facility constructed to address overcrowding at Stockton Asylum. NSH was once self-sufficient, with its own dairy and poultry ranches, vegetable gardens, orchards, and other farming operations. For more than 120 years, NSH's primary patient population included individuals who had been civilly committed, individuals who were developmentally disabled and could not be maintained in a less restrictive environment, and juveniles who required long-term inpatient psychiatric treatment unavailable in their county. Although built for 500 patients, the census peaked in 1960, with more than 5,000 individuals receiving treatment. At the time of this writing, the NSH census was 1,283.

From the 1960s through the 1990s, the national movement for deinstitutionalization of individuals with mental disorders resulted in numerous discharges and a dwindling patient population in the California state hospital system. At one point during the mid-1990s, there were serious concerns that NSH might close as the number of occupied beds was greatly diminished. During this same period, a phenomenon known as "criminalization of the mentally ill" was occurring, in which patients with mental disorders living in the community committed a range of criminal offenses that resulted in their entry into the criminal justice system. Because various legal statutes required involuntary psychiatric hospitalization of offenders with mental illness, an increase in forensic psychiatric beds for this rising forensic population in California was needed. One answer to this dilemma involved converting many of NSH's prior civil commitment beds to forensic beds. In 1998, a Secure Treatment Area (STA) was established at NSH with the plan to house all forensic patients in this area. This STA conversion, which was designed to be physically separate from the remaining civil commitment beds, included the construction of a razor wire fence around its perimeter and a sally-port security entrance manned by hospital police.

With the construction of the STA, NSH became primarily a forensic hospital, although the staff had previously treated a very different patient population. Frank Turlington, the NSH Executive Director at that time, recognized that the

executive team and his hospital staff required training on how to best treat this
new patient population. As a result, NSH contracted with Dr. Yarvis, the forensic
psychiatry division chief at UC Davis, to provide both education on forensic issues to NSH staff and general forensic consultation on issues related to the transition to a facility serving mostly forensic patients.

In October of 1998, Dr. Charles Scott joined the UC Davis forensic psychiatry division as the forensic fellowship training director. The contract between
NSH and UC Davis expanded to include his services as the site supervisor for
forensic psychiatry fellows and case consultant to the treatment teams and hospital executive team. Over the next 2 years, both agencies involved in the collaboration recognized the need for research to best address questions on the safe
management and effective treatment of this relatively new population. In 2001,
Dr. Barbara McDermott was recruited as a research director by UC Davis to serve
in this important role.

THE PROCESS INVOLVED IN SETTING IT UP

The first step in setting up the collaboration was defining the amount of time
and requested scope of work to be delivered; NSH would fund this through a financial agreement with the UC Davis Department of Psychiatry and Behavioral
Services. The initial scope of work included a list of specific forensic training sessions to be delivered by Dr. Yarvis to the hospital staff (i.e., mental health staff,
nursing staff, hospital police, etc.) and consultative time to the executive director
and executive team.

Second, once the scope of work and cost of funded time were agreed on, each
agency had its own contract office review the document to ensure compliance
with each agency's relevant policies. Because the UC system has additional financial overhead costs beyond payment of faculty to deliver the services, educating
the NSH executive director and team about these additional costs was critical in
answering any questions that might have deterred signing of the contract.

Third, the contract expanded over time to include on-site training and case
consultation by Dr. Charles Scott and delivery of services by UC Davis forensic
psychiatry fellows. Dr. Scott's case consultation involved review of high-risk or
high-profile cases identified by the medical director and utilized the forensic
psychiatry fellows to assist with conducting case reviews, writing consultative
reports, and presenting findings to treatment teams. With the addition of both
Dr. Scott and two forensic psychiatry fellows, the financial contribution by NSH
for the contracted services increased. In 2000, a Forensic Visiting Scholars program was created, with a separate line item funding to support training from
national and international experts on the assessment and treatment of forensic
offenders. The contract with NSH funded the visiting scholar speaker fee, travel,
and cost of the off-site auditorium. In 2002, Dr. Yarvis retired and Dr. Scott's
role and committed time expanded to include responsibility for hospital-wide
training.

Once core forensic training sessions were developed by Dr. Scott and provided to NSH for more than a decade, Dr. Katherine Warburton, the DSH Medical Director, recognized that similar training would likely benefit the other four state hospitals. To accomplish that goal, DSH entered into a separate contractual agreement with UC Davis in 2016. This separate contract funded Dr. Scott to develop and provide statewide training on core concepts in treating forensic patients This training was provided through a WebEx seminar so that all hospitals were educated on emerging and important issues. An associated series of core competency examinations was developed so attendees could demonstrate their proficiency achieved from delivered training. These examinations were voluntary only and not required for credentialing of any staff at any of the forensic facilities. Staff could choose which, if any, of the examinations they wished to take from those topic areas relevant to their specific work. Staff were offered continued educational credits for attending the seminar, whether or not they took the examination. The performance on the examination (i.e., pass or fail) had no adverse impact on performance appraisals. However, individuals who passed the examination could include this positive outcome in their training file, add it to their curriculum vitae, and use it to establish their qualifications when testifying in court. The percentage of attendees who took each examination varied widely according to the particular topic, with a range of 20–50% of attendees signing up to take an examination.

A research program was considered crucial as the hospital transitioned from treating civilly to forensically committed patients. NSH agreed to fund a forensic research director who would be recruited and employed by UC Davis but assigned on site at NSH. The research conducted at NSH was mandated to be forensically relevant but also clinically applicable to inform the hospital administration about issues pertinent to treating justice-involved patients. All studies were required to inform the mission of the hospital: the treatment, assessment, and release of offenders with a major mental disorder.

The development of the research program was the responsibility of the research director, who was recruited specifically for this position. The negotiation for the research program included a commitment from the hospital to establish a research unit designed exclusively for conducting studies with forensic patients. Existing hospital staff were selected specifically for this unit, which was staffed at a higher level than most units. A hospital-wide announcement of positions on this newly developed research unit was disseminated, and interested staff volunteered to be interviewed for this unit. The selection panel consisted of two forensic psychiatrists and one forensic psychologist from the University of California, Davis, the NSH Medical Director, the NSH Associate Medical Director, the NSH Chief of Social Work, and the NSH Chief of Rehabilitation Services. The research unit included two complete treatment teams, with each team consisting of a psychiatrist, psychologist, social worker, and rehabilitation therapist. Nursing staff was enhanced as well, and all staff agreed to participate in all structured research programs as a condition of being assigned to this unit. Weekly meetings were held with research staff, which included all treatment providers. These meetings were designed to provide consistent feedback about the status of research endeavors.

Additionally, the contract between UC Davis and NSH provided funding for a variety of UC Davis faculty and staff. At the initiation of the research program, the contract included funding for the research director, one part-time psychologist, and three research assistants. Napa agreed to provide one research analyst and an office technician to assist in the management of the data and the technical aspects of the program. The nature of the contract has evolved over the 18 years that it has been in effect, which will be described later.

Two key components of a successful contractual collaboration have included ongoing feedback on accomplishments of each program as well as monitoring of the contract and establishing when and how the contracts are renegotiated. Progress monitoring has been provided through ongoing meetings between the forensic division chief with the hospital executive director (initially weekly then decreasing to monthly); annual visits and meetings of the Department Chair to NSH, which included meeting with the executive team to ensure contract compliance and satisfaction; monthly meetings between the research director and the executive policy team at NSH; and in-person meetings between the NSH hospital executive team and key leadership from UC Davis when contracts are renegotiated. In general, the contract has included a clause specifying a time frame within which either party can exercise the right to terminate the contract, though that has never occurred to date. However, both sides set agreed-upon dates for contract renegotiation because this allows revisions as needed to address emerging concerns or changes in the budget. All contracts are typically set for 2 or 3 years. Having contracts renewed on an annual basis would require a substantial amount of administrative time that is probably unnecessary; it would also limit effective long-term planning and stability.

WHO IS INVOLVED

The individuals involved in the contract and the leadership responsibilities have changed over time. The initial leadership collaboration was led by Dr. Richard Yarvis from UC Davis and Frank Turlington, the executive director of NSH. Dr. Yarvis was funded approximately 0.4 full-time equivalents (FTE) to develop and implement on-site training and consultation to the executive team. In 1998, Dr. Charles Scott was added to the funded contract and was initially funded 0.2 FTE, which was increased to 0.4 FTE by 2000. Two forensic psychiatry fellows were initially assigned to NSH as a training site (one per 6-month rotation), and NSH provided salary support for 1.0 FTE forensic psychiatry fellow (covering both 6-month rotations). As the fellowship program grew larger and more established, NSH provided additional salary support for forensic psychiatry fellows. The contract expanded further with the addition of Dr. Barbara McDermott in 2001, as research director at NSH. The contract funded the research director position at 1.0 FTE but, as noted previously, also funded additional research personnel.

Key duties of forensic psychiatry division chief (initially led by Dr. Yarvis until 2002 and then by Dr. Scott since then) have been to develop a scope of work that evolves with needs of the organization, provide consultations as requested to members of the NSH executive team, supervise the forensic psychiatry fellows on their case consultations, serve as site supervisor for fellowship training, monitor contract compliance, regularly check in with leadership at both NSH and DSH to assess contract satisfaction and adjust as needed, review educational surveys of training provided on site and through statewide seminars, complete necessary paperwork for ACGME accreditation relevant to training site, establish acceptable time commitment for requested services, and work with the UC Davis Chairman and its Chief Financial Officer to develop and monitor the contract in compliance with university policies. Key duties of NSH and subsequently DSH leadership have been to clearly define their desired scope of work, identify state contractual requirements, make payments as scheduled and immediately alert UC Davis if any budgetary changes adversely impact payment, and provide appropriate onsite resources for delivery of services. Such resources have included adequate office space for faculty, assigned fellows, and research assistants; security clearances for access to hospital and administrative buildings; computers with access to relevant databases to perform work; and an identified on-site coordinator to address questions or concerns that may arise.

WHAT SERVICES ARE DELIVERED

Three primary services have been delivered since the inception of the collaboration in 1998. These are (1) consultation and on-site forensic evaluations, (2) education and training of staff at DSH facilities, and (3) research on issues relevant to treatment and management of forensic patients.

Consultation and On-Site Forensic Evaluations

Forensic consultations to member of the executive team have included general recommendations for providing forensic services to DSH facilities as well as case-specific recommendations. Case-specific consultations typically involve risk assessment of general recidivism or sexual recidivism if released, malingering of symptoms, management of aggression or violence within the facility, and trial competency restoration status. In 1998, Dr. Scott became responsible for providing second-opinion consultations for Medical Director Dr. Jeffrey Zwerin and treatment teams. This consultation was conducted utilizing the forensic psychiatry fellows with supervision provided by Dr. Scott. During the first 10 years of the contract, these consultations involved assigning a forensic psychiatry fellow to a specific case. The fellow conducted a detailed review of records and a forensic psychiatric evaluation with relevant testing and/or risk assessments. A case conference was held at which the findings and recommendation were presented to the treatment team by the UC Davis fellow. With changing priorities of the hospital, the fellows' scope of work has been modified and now includes three key roles: (1)

conducting evaluations to determine if an individual found IST has been restored to competency, (2) conducting violence and sexual risk assessments in consultation with the medical director and treatment teams, and (3) conducting forensic quality review of individuals found NGRI to help identify barriers for potential release.

In addition, when the DSH facilities were under a period of court monitoring, Dr. McDermott and Dr. Scott met with the court monitors to assist the hospital in answering any specific questions requiring more forensic expertise and to assist in the reasonable implementation of new requirements of the consent decree. This court monitoring evolved from a 2002 Civil Rights of Institutionalized Persons Act (CRIPA) investigation against Metropolitan State Hospital that focused on the care and treatment provided to the facility's child and adolescent patients. This investigation was subsequently extended to examine the care and treatment also provided to adult patients at this facility. In a proactive response to any potential investigations into other facilities, DSH retained forensic mental health experts to provide systemic recommendations on both the assessment and treatment of all DSH patients.

Education and Staff Training

The education and training services delivered through the collaboration between NSH and DSH have evolved over the 20 years that it has been in place. During the first year (1998–1999), Dr. Yarvis provided hospital-wide training on general issues related to working in a forensic facility. After Dr. Yarvis's retirement in 2002, Dr. Scott assumed responsibility for the training of hospital personnel. These training sessions have provided educational credits for physicians, psychologists, social workers, and nursing staff. The training sessions have been provided on site, typically during the noon lunch hour. Lunch was not provided by hospital administration but staff were encouraged to bring their own lunch, leading to this training series being coined the "brown bag" lecture series. For some key topics during the course of this collaboration, hospital leadership mandated the training, with sign-in sheets and attendance documented. The mandatory attendance was tracked by supervisors, and mandatory presentations were presented on numerous occasions and on different shifts to ensure compliance. Mandatory topics included training sessions related to violence risk assessment and management of aggression, forensic report writing and testimony, and the impact of the *Diagnostic and Statistical Manual-Fifth Edition* on the assessment of forensic patients. Attendance was substantially increased for those training sessions deemed mandatory by hospital administration. Continuing education credits were provided for all training sessions, regardless of whether or not administration required the training. A sample of training topics are included in Box 6.1.

Training needs were also adapted to hospital needs. For example, with increasing concerns about aggression by patients toward other patients and staff, mandatory hospital training on this topic was provided to all hospital personnel. This training

Box 6.1

FORENSIC LECTURE TOPICS FOR HOSPITAL TRAINING

Violence risk assessment
  Sexual violence risk assessment
  Assessment of malingering
  Competency to stand trial
  Not guilty by reason of insanity
  Mentally disordered offender
  Mental health malpractice
  Aggression reduction training
  Psychiatric civil commitment
  Involuntary medication treatment and forensic offenders
  Expert witness testimony
  Principles of forensic report writing

was based on a study of aggression and violence at the NSH facility and therefore very relevant to the treatment providers.

After approximately 15 years, DSH leadership decided that it would be important to export the forensic lecture training series offered by Dr. Scott to all DSH facilities. To accomplish this, a separate contract was initiated by DSH for Dr. Scott to provide training on forensic topics to all five state hospitals through a WebEx seminar broadcast from DSH headquarters in Sacramento. These training sessions provided continuing professional education credits and an examination that attendees could access online immediately after the WebEx presentation. In addition, this DSH contract funded Dr. Scott to provide training at specific DSH facilities as needed. All professional disciplines (psychiatry, psychology, social work, nursing staff, and rehabilitation staff) were invited to attend these training sessions, and continuing education credits were provided for psychiatry and psychology.

Research

The research program evolved over the years. The initial research plan involved staffing a research/treatment unit with the ability to conduct multiple studies with forensic patients in addition to providing forensically relevant treatment. Patients would consent to participate in research and transfer to this unit for a specific period of time. Because the mission of most forensic facilities, at least in part, is the reduction of violence, the first study for which we sought approval was longitudinal and designed to collect data on violence risk and factors associated with violence. The research plan was to follow the patient into the community to evaluate which of the factors were related to outcome and which were associated with release decisions. Pitfalls of that research design will be discussed later. Early on, it became apparent that using research data to determine if the assessments conducted were associated with institutional aggression became a critical area of concern for the administration. Concerns about escalating rates of aggression had become a pressing matter. Data were collected to evaluate this issue, resulting in several publications (McDermott, Dualan, & Scott, 2011; McDermott, Edens, Quanbeck, Busse, & Scott, 2008; McDermott, Quanbeck, Busse, Yastro, & Scott, 2008; Quanbeck et al., 2007). More importantly, clinical procedures were modified as a result of this research to include a brief assessment of violence risk on admission. Later in the program, examining issues associated with patients found IST became critical. A research procedure was developed to evaluate characteristics of patients admitted as IST, which ultimately became a mandated clinical procedure. The data collected from this procedure have been used to make numerous policy and statutory changes—and have also resulted in publications (McDermott, Newman, Meyer, Scott, & Warburton, 2017; McDermott, Warburton, & Auletta-Young, 2019).

Who Is Served

Although many different groups benefit from the collaboration, the primary group ultimately served are the patients treated by the California DSH. Patients are better served through this collaboration by providing training to staff to improve assessment and treatment, recruiting fellows to stay on staff at the completion of their fellowship, educating leadership about implementation of policies and procedures likely to assist in improvement, and conducting research to identify additional interventions and treatment special to this population. The research in particular has been used to provide evidence for best practices or to pilot procedures that ultimately have resulted in modifications to clinical practice. Moreover, the data informed DSH and the administration about the characteristics of patients admitted as IST. This knowledge resulted in the implementation of a pretrial diversion program to address the needs of this specific group of patients. Without the collaborative relationship between DSH and UC Davis, these programmatic changes would not have occurred.

HOW THE COLLABORATION FUNCTIONS

In this section, we discuss in more detail how the various tasks involved in this collaboration are actually carried out.

Consultation and Case Reviews

The forensic consultations conducted at NSH are provided by the forensic psychiatry fellows. Key components necessary to train and supervise the assigned forensic psychiatry fellows include the following:

- A UC Davis and NSH site supervisors responsible for the selection and supervision of case consultations are identified. Dr. Barbara McDermott is the site supervisor responsible for providing the training and oversight on specific assessment instruments for NSH case evaluations and consultations.
- The site supervisors meet weekly with the fellows to review current assignments and track their progress. At the beginning of the training year, the site supervisors observe the fellows interview patients so the supervisors can teach and provide feedback on skills for forensic interviewing. Detailed training is also provided to the fellows on forensic report writing by the site supervisors.
- The fellows' reports are reviewed by both the UC Davis and DSH site supervisors before submission to the Medical Director. When fellows are assigned to conduct trial competency evaluations, their reports are typically reviewed and submitted within 2 working days of the evaluation. This rapid turnaround is important because there is a waiting list for individuals to enter the DSH system, and minimizing any delays is critical to support the hospital's mission.
- The UC Davis site director periodically meets with the Chief of Staff and Medical Director to ensure their hospital needs are being appropriately addressed through these case consultations.
- The fellows' performance is reviewed through weekly monitoring of their work progress, through evaluations by all three site supervisors, and by NSH staff who provide feedback on questionnaires sent to them.

Training of Staff

When training was provided only at NSH, the training topics were selected based on needs identified by Dr. Charles Scott and the NSH executive team. As described earlier, some selected training topics were mandatory for staff to attend while others were voluntary. The administration sent hospital-wide notices and worked with division chiefs and supervisors to ensure that all staff were aware of which training sessions were mandatory. Once the training topics were selected, a list of training dates and times was selected and coordination with the hospital continuing medical education (CME) was initiated. An important aspect of this didactic training relationship is encouraging as many disciplines to attend training as possible. This is facilitated by working with the organization to determine what requirements are necessary to authorize continuing educational credits for each discipline. The UC Davis psychiatrist contracted to provide the training is responsible for completing the relevant training forms and submitting them to the hospital CME office. The CME office is responsible for organizing a post-training survey, tabulating the survey results, and providing these results to the UC Davis educator.

A similar process was developed for Dr. Scott's DSH statewide training. An additional component, however, is DSH's responsibility to ensure adequate technical support so the WebEx presentations are received by each facility. Like the NSH presentations, each of the WebEx presentations is followed by a survey that includes detailed questions about the impact and effectiveness of the presenter and presentation. In contrast to the local hospital training sessions, this DSH statewide training also provided a series of voluntary topic-specific competency examinations offered to all attendees of this statewide WebEx presentation.

Research

Research topics were based entirely on the mission of the hospital, with certain areas of study identified as more critical over time. One pressing issue early in the contract was understanding the rates of institutional violence. Many research studies were designed to assist the hospital administration in developing programs to address the issue of inpatient aggression. Areas of study were developed in consultation with this administration. Although the contract evolved to a statewide endeavor, this communication regarding priorities was and continues to be a major component in the success and continued funding of the research program.

Having the research staff based at the hospital also has been critical to the success of the program. The research director was funded as a full-time position with the expectation that this individual would maintain offices at NSH. All research staff hired by UC Davis on this contract were based at NSH. Although this arrangement is likely atypical in state agency–university collaborations, it has been a key component to the success of the collaborative research process. One major strength is that having a visible presence on a daily basis at the hospital allowed the research program to become an integral part of the hospital's functioning. Moreover, a consistent physical presence allowed the research staff to be included in relevant committees developed to inform policy decisions. The research director has been included in multiple committees developed to assess relevant problems. For example, a committee that included the research director was formed in 2007 to discuss the problem of increasing IST admissions. As a result of this committee's work, a screening procedure was piloted by the research division to gather data on the characteristics of the IST admissions. This pilot procedure became clinical policy and resulted in almost 10 years of structured data-gathering with these patients. This likely would not have occurred if the research staff were not based at the hospital.

The Expectations and Agreements That Have Worked Best

The areas of collaboration that have worked best involve tailoring the presentations to key learning gaps for hospital staff and identifying relevant emergent topics. For example, when key court decisions relevant to the treatment of hospital patients are released, Dr. Scott summarizes the case and implications for the hospital administration and treating staff. As noted earlier, the statewide DSH WebEx training sessions also offer voluntary core competency tests that have been useful in illustrating material learned and highlighting other areas of deficit for those staff who choose to take the examination. Case consultations have proved most effective when team members feel included in the process and their input is recognized. During the first decade of this collaboration, the case consultations focused on high-risk cases that required detailed and often exhaustive, time-consuming record reviews. This process raised some concerns about "bang for the buck" regarding the amount of time required for what seemed like relatively few deliverables. Because the hospital needed more timely evaluations (e.g., competency to stand trial evaluations), the expectations for the fellows changed to include a mix of both briefer competency evaluation and more in-depth risk assessments. This combination has seemed to work best for meeting the needs of both the contracting organization and fellowship training.

As noted previously, having the research based at the hospital was key to the success of the program. This day-to-day contact allowed the research program to be woven into the fabric of the hospital. The research director and research staff became a part of the hospital's functioning, which might not have happened if the staff had been based primarily at the university. Another key component that has worked exceedingly well is the communication of research results and, more importantly, communication regarding the needs of the system, which initially was focused on NSH but subsequently expanded to include the entire state hospital system. Research results were communicated in a variety of ways, including meetings with administrative staff. Presentations to the staff at the hospital were scheduled on a regular basis, so treatment providers were informed of results and suggestions for best practices. Eventually, presenting the results of the research at the yearly Forensic Visiting Scholars program was instrumental in disseminating these results. In 2007, NSH made several changes to its forensic services, including hiring a forensically trained psychiatrist, Dr. Katherine Warburton, as the Chief of Forensic Services, a newly developed division. Formerly, this division focused on liaison between the hospital and community, primarily associated with the release of long-term patients, and was directed by a social worker. With a forensic psychiatrist appointed as chief, the role expanded to include all issues relevant to the treatment and management of forensic patients. As a forensic psychiatrist, Dr. Warburton attended forensic conferences and acquired a keen understanding of the issues facing forensic hospitals. More importantly, because of her training, she also was aware of the benefits of using data to promote policy change. The strength of the relationship between this position and the UC Davis personnel was critical. The bidirectional nature of the relationship has been key to the success of the research program and has aided the system in using data to make significant changes. An example is the IST admission screening, developed by the research division to answer a question asked by Dr. Warburton: Is the length of stay longer at NSH than at other facilities because of the number of patients who are malingering? The ability to pose these questions and obtain responses based on data has been critical and perhaps best characterized as a partnership rather than a service.

Because of the substantial utility of having data to drive policy decisions (such as, for example, statutory changes requiring that forensic evaluators receive training), a public policy rotation was implemented as a pilot in 2015–2016 with a fellow funded by an external agency that had expressed interest in a public policy rotation. In addition to his general forensic training, this individual spent 1 day per week in the state office under the supervision of Dr. Katherine Warburton, who was serving as both medical director and the director of clinical operations for DSH. During his rotation, the fellow developed and administered a survey assessing an emerging issue that state hospitals were facing: increasing numbers of IST commitments. This research led to a publication (Warburton, McDermott, Gale, & Stahl, 2020) and, more importantly, provided an opportunity for California to join in the conversation about a national problem. Because of the success of this pilot, funding was provided by DSH for an additional forensic fellow to focus on public policy issues. The current fellows are now working on a project critical to DSH involving understanding the functioning of jail-based restoration of trial competency.

The Expectations and Agreements That Have Not Worked Well

After NSH became mostly a forensic facility, staff were subpoenaed to court but had limited skill in providing expert testimony. Early during the relationship, Dr. Scott established a mock trial experience for the hospital, with hospital staff testifying in front of a large group of their peers. Although the use of mock trials is a critical component in a forensic psychiatry fellowship program, non-forensically trained staff were not prepared for the intensity and rigor of such mock cross examinations. In fact, this training experience seemed to resemble being attacked publicly in a Roman coliseum, which could never be pleasurable or enhance learning. As a result, a certain anxiety and/or fear about participating in this training experience developed and did not foster a positive relationship between UC Davis faculty and NSH staff. To address this error, Dr. Scott and hospital leadership met to create an alternate experience to improve testimony skills, which the hospital recognized was greatly needed. Under a revised model, a decision was made to only hold mock testimony examinations in front of small groups, such as the staff's own treatment team, rather than larger fora. Before any small-group mock testimony training sessions were conducted, Dr. Scott first provided a hospital-wide training regarding the specific goals of the mock trial experience, with the fellows serving as role models under mock direct and cross-examination. A preparation checklist was provided that would help members prepare for the smaller testimony training experience. This "checklist" included instructions for the individual to list their background and training, their occupational duties and experience, the specific legal issue on the case selected for mock trial testimony, a clear forensic opinion about their conclusion on the legal opinion, and the need to have specific evidence to support the opinion. In addition, CMEs were also organized for this mock trial experience using this much smaller group format. Before each mock trial training experience, Dr. Scott reviews the steps on how the mock trial will proceed, including specific questions that will be asked on direct and cross-examination. To help decrease any anxiety staff may experience "on the witness stand," Dr. Scott takes frequent breaks to provide feedback and gather input from the small group.

Similarly, during the initial few years of the contract, Dr. Scott and the fellows met with the treatment teams after lengthy large consultations in high-profile or high-risk cases. At times, the UC Davis consultation team (i.e., forensic fellow and Dr. Scott) uncovered a great deal of information not known by the treatment team or reached a significantly different opinion on the diagnosis and/or risk assessment. When meeting as a large group to present findings, there were situations in which treatment team members were exposed to strikingly different conclusions from the UC Davis consultants, which led to understandably uncomfortable if not embarrassing situations. To minimize the impact on treating providers, the UC Davis fellow and Dr. Scott both tried to identify any possible disagreements early in the consultative process and sought input from the treatment team before any final diagnoses or recommendations were provided. When presenting the case consultations, the UC Davis team might have differed with the findings of the treatment team, but we provided detailed evidence to support our conclusions, cited specific examples from the records, and provided relevant research and literature consistent with our findings.

Although Dr. Yarvis and the NSH administration were well-intentioned, the most problematic component of the research plan involved designating a research unit as the primary site for conducting forensically relevant research. One of the most important roles in the treatment of patients found dangerous because of their mental disorder is managing the symptoms of the mental disorder that led to their offense. Treating a mental disorder requires assessing the patient to determine the nature of the mental disorder and identifying those factors that are most likely to increase—or decrease—their risk of violence. At the opening of the research unit, Napa was organized into treatment-specific units. Certain units were co-ed (there were no all-female units at the time of this study), and others were identified as "open" units, meaning that the doors to the unit were unlocked during certain times of day. These patients were typically more stable and were free to leave at any point during the permitted hours—and were not required to have a particular destination when doing so. The research unit was designed as a locked unit in order to recruit a range of patients (not just those who were closer to discharge). It also was intentionally designed to be co-ed because of the paucity of research with female offenders. Unfortunately, the co-ed component limited the types of men who could be admitted to this unit for safety reasons. Additionally, patients on the open units were highly unlikely to consent to participate because of the requirement that they transfer to a locked unit. Moreover, in a long-term hospital, patients often develop relationships with their treatment teams, feel they are making progress in their treatment, and are hesitant to consent to a transfer to another team. On multiple occasions, patients would participate in the lengthy consenting process and withdraw consent after discussing the decision with their treatment providers. Eventually, we were able to obtain more representative samples by recruiting participants from the open units and later from all-male locked units without the requirement of transfer to the research unit to obtain such samples. The lesson learned: when designing research in a long-term facility, don't develop a designated research unit or any system of participation that would limit the representativeness of your sample. Although we were able to overcome this hurdle by modifying the research procedures to not require transfer to the designated research unit, the concept of a single research unit in a long-term hospital is not workable when researchers wish to engage participants from across different units.

Significant Changes Since It Began

From a case consultative perspective, the most significant change has been the transition from having fellows conducting primarily lengthier risk assessments to conducting more short-term competency evaluations. In addition, previous practice involved assigning only one fellow to rotate through NSH at a time. Fellows were clear in their feedback that they wished to rotate on site together, so Dr. Scott reworked the schedule to allow all fellows providing services to NSH to be present on the same 2 days each week. The major training change has been the shift of Dr. Scott's forensic didactic series from on site at NSH to a WebEx seminar that delivers the lectures to all five DSH facilities from DSH headquarters in Sacramento.

Changes in the Research Contract

The collaboration between the state hospital system and UC Davis has spanned various challenges. Two of the most important, which we discuss in this section, have been changes in leadership (both in NSH and DSH) and changes in the fiscal climate.

CHANGES IN LEADERSHIP

Although the initial contract was with one of the state hospitals (NSH), all contracts were approved at the state level and all hospitals reported to the state administration. At the time of the initial contracts, the state department managing the long-term state hospital system was the DMH. The organizational structure included one commissioner and several deputy commissioners—one of whom was the deputy commissioner of long-term care (the state hospital system). The system reorganized in 2012, and various functions were assigned to other departments or to counties. With the accompanying reorganization of the system, a separate division was created to oversee the clinical operations of the hospital system. Dr. Warburton, appointed to oversee the clinical operations, began her administrative career at NSH and used data collected in the research at Napa to inform various policy decisions. Because of this, a new 3-year contract was negotiated with DSH to replicate many of the studies conducted at NSH to the other four hospitals. Eight research assistants were included in this contract to provide technical support for this expanded research mission.

Changes in Fiscal Climate

Changes in the fiscal climate necessitated multiple revisions to the research portion of the contract, with positions removed with each subsequent 3-year renewal to reduce costs. The final revision occurred in 2009, reducing research personnel to the research director, one UC Davis-funded research assistant, and one NSH-funded office technician. Although an active research program was maintained, many of the procedures developed as pilot studies had been integrated into clinical practice, and data were collected from these clinical procedures.

Contractual Details

At the time this chapter was written, there were three main contracts for services: one contract involving services delivered by Dr. Scott at NSH and the forensic psychiatry fellows, a second for Dr. Scott's training services for DSH, and a third for Dr. McDermott's responsibility in overseeing statewide DSH research activities. Key components of all contracts are the listing of agencies entering the agreement, terms of when the contract starts and ends, maximum amount of financial payment authorized by the contract, and specific terms and conditions for the work to be performed. A specific scope of work for all parties was attached to the contract. The scope of work details the service location, service hours, key personnel delivering the services, university responsibilities, and specific services to be delivered. The state's responsibilities were also delineated and included the right to conduct quality assurance of the delivered services, financial audits, monitoring and evaluation of services delivered, and review of university financial records relevant to the contract. A separate exhibit outlining the specific budget, justification of the budget, invoice elements, and university terms and conditions was also attached to the contract. A listing of specific lectures and training sessions are part of the services agreement for the forensic training at the statewide level with DSH including a contractual requirement for Dr. Scott to develop a statewide competency curriculum and examination program. Likewise, duties specific to Dr. Scott's consulting to both NSH and DSH were identified. These included consulting on high-risk cases, describing forensic issues relevant to the management of patients, and coordinating with the DSH medical director to create a national annual forensic forum.

LESSONS LEARNED AND IMPLICATIONS

The collaboration described in this chapter has been long-standing and valuable. It has also been informative, as we discuss in this section.

Forensic Case Consultation: Lessons Learned

Four key lessons on conducting forensic case consultations have been learned from the two decades of this collaboration. First, identifying the opinions of and personal investment in the case of treatment team providers is important to minimize and manage conflicts, either between team members or between the team and the consultant. Second, before any final opinion is rendered (either verbally or in writing), the consultant should clearly and publicly ask team members for their input and reasons for their opinions. By doing this, the consultant can more diplomatically introduce different opinions without alienating team members. Third, the UC Davis consultant should produce a written report as soon as possible after the case consultation to maintain consultative momentum and to show respect for the patient and treatment team. Fourth, the forensic consultant should assist the hospital in selecting those cases in which a forensic consultation might actually make a difference. If an extensive consultation is unlikely to change the outcome, then the facility may not realize any benefit from the consultation—and overlook those cases in which a second opinion might make a difference. Working with the forensic office, medical director, or other members of the executive team can help identify cases needing an academic level of forensic consultation and clearly delineate the referral questions.

Forensic Didactic Training: Lessons Learned

Lessons learned in providing forensic didactic training are also clear. We would describe the key lessons as follows:

- When creating a training curriculum, survey both administration and staff to help develop a list of relevant topics;
- Provide continuing educational credits to encourage attendance;
- Work with administration to select key training sessions as "mandatory";
- Have administration visibly present at the actual training during the initial years of collaboration to publicly demonstrate their commitment to and support for the training;
- Combine training with detailed handouts and post-presentation knowledge appraisal so attendees can apply and test their knowledge;
- Conduct post-training surveys to receive feedback on training provided;

- Be prepared for some very challenging, even confrontational, feedback from participants who resent having to attend mandatory training sessions—always handle such responses with professionalism and strive to find respectful areas of agreement and disagreement;
- Wherever possible, include practical case vignettes that parallel those challenging cases currently faced by hospital staff.
- Select a time and place convenient for the staff, not the presenter; and
- Consider presenting with a staff member to increase the sense of shared responsibility and buy-in from other staff members.

Lessons from the Research Program

The research program has provided several important lessons. We discuss these lessons in this section.

LESSONS ABOUT IRB APPROVAL

Because the research was a collaborative process between a University and a state agency, both had established processes for approving human subject research. At UC Davis, institutional review board (IRB) approval is required before the initiation of any research involving human subjects. No UC Davis employee is permitted to engage in human subject research without IRB approval. In California, any research conducted with individuals under the jurisdiction of the Department of Health and Human Services (DHHS) requires approval by the California Committee for the Protection of Human Subjects (CPHS). DSH (and formerly the Department of Mental Health) is governed by DHHS, so any studies conducted with these patients requires CPHS approval. UC Davis and CPHS had slightly different formats for submitting an application to conduct research involving human participants, including different formats for consent forms. This resulted in the need for two separate consent forms for the same study (although, as the study progressed, both agencies agreed to the language on a single consent form). One important lesson is that it is possible to get agreement between two regulatory bodies: the state and university IRBs. In recent years, the UC IRB has entered into "reliance" agreements with CPHS, wherein UCD relies on the approval of CPHS (CPHS requires as policy that if state patients participate in research, then CPHS must be the primary IRB). In fact, the new Common Rule will require a single IRB in January 2020 for federally funded research efforts.

In 1981, the Code of Federal Regulations, Title 45, Part 46 (45 CFR 46), also called the Common Rule, was enacted. It outlines the requisite procedures for conducting federally funded research. When strictly interpreted, these regulations only apply to federally funded research or research regulated by a federal agency (e.g., the Food and Drug Administration). In practice, most IRBs and human subject committees follow the guidelines set forth in the Common Rule. In these regulations, additional protections are provided for certain classes of participants

(Subparts B [pregnant women, human fetuses, neonates], C [prisoners], and D [children]), with specific regulations for each class. According to these regulations, the definition of a prisoner included any individual committed to a penal institution via a criminal or civil court, or any institution to which these individuals were sent in lieu of incarceration. Research involving prisoners must be of minimal risk and limited to four areas of study:

1. study of the possible causes, effects, and processes of incarceration, and of criminal behavior;
2. study of prisons as institutional structures or of prisoners as incarcerated persons;
3. research on conditions particularly affecting prisoners as a class; and
4. research on practices, both innovative and accepted, which have the intent and reasonable probability of improving the health or well-being of the subject.

Most importantly, release decisions could not be affected in any way by participation in research. Because the mission of most forensic facilities, at least in part, is the reduction of violence, the first study for which we sought approval was a longitudinal study designed to collect data on violence risk and factors associated with violence. The research plan was to follow the patient into the community to evaluate which of the assessments, if any, were related to outcome, and which, if any, were associated with release decisions. At the time of the initial approval for this study, the UC Davis IRB did not consider the patients at DSH-Napa to meet the federal definition of a prisoner and, as such, did not require that the study meet the additional guidelines for research with prisoners. This was not true for CPHS. This committee required that the study be modified so that data collected as part of the research would not be considered in release decision-making. The committee's interpretation of the Common Rule was that data collected for research purposes could not be used in making release decisions, not that participation in research could not be considered in making release decisions or recommendations. Hence the second lesson: understand the guidelines for conducting research in the specific population you are studying. Forensic patients are now uniformly considered to be in this class and require additional research protections. Probationers and parolees are typically included in this definition as well, as are other justice-involved individuals.

Lessons About Informed Consent

Because all of the participants were committed to DSH-Napa as a result of a major mental disorder, CPHS also required an assessment of capacity to provide consent. The assessment selected (the MacArthur Competence Assessment Tool for Consent to Clinical Research [MacCAT-CR]) provided valuable information and resulted in a publication (McDermott, Gerbasi, Quanbeck, & Scott, 2005) that informed the discussion about the capacity of individuals with major mental disorders to provide informed consent. However, the consenting process required a minimum of 45 minutes, in part because of this capacity assessment. It was not uncommon for the consenting process to require 2 hours. Moreover, whenever research is conducted on individuals with major mental disorders, a periodic evaluation of consent is critical. More than one individual had to be withdrawn from the study because of psychiatric decompensation leading to an inability to provide continued informed consent. Lesson learned: when you are required to use two unique consent forms, don't select a capacity assessment that mirrors the consent forms. Guidelines do not require such a lengthy assessment, and, at the time of this writing, the federal guidelines do not consider individuals with a serious mental disorder to be a protected class. IRBs, however, generally require a capacity assessment for participants who are either seriously mentally ill or economically disadvantaged and always require an assessment of capacity in participants who are likely to have cognitive deficits.

CONCLUSION

The collaboration between UC Davis and DSH has spanned two decades. It has been maintained through remarkably austere economic times and has flourished in recent years as the breadth of the contract has expanded to cover the entire California hospital system. The key components of this remarkable collaboration have involved identifying relevant and changing needs of a large forensic hospital system and adjusting to meet those needs, delivering practical rather than esoteric training, providing consultations that assist in solving diagnostic and legal challenges, developing and designing research protocols that have utility for the system, and maintaining a close and collaborative relationship with administration.

This collaboration has been largely successful because of the mutual respect that both agencies have developed since its inception in 1998, with both sides giving to and benefiting from each other. In the wise and paraphrased words of the Dalai Lama, mutual respect is essential for creating a harmonious relationship between two groups.

REFERENCES

California Department of State Hospitals. (2019). Mission Statement. https://www.dsh. ca.gov/About_Us/index.html

McDermott, B. E., Dualan, I. V., & Scott, C. L. (2011). The predictive ability of the Classification of Violence Risk (COVR) in a forensic psychiatric hospital. *Psychiatric Services, 62*, 430–433. doi:10.1176/ps.62.4.pss6204_0430

McDermott, B. E., Edens, J. F., Quanbeck, C. D., Busse, D., & Scott, C. L. (2008). Examining the role of static and dynamic risk factors in the prediction of inpatient violence: Variable- and person-focused analyses. *Law and Human Behavior, 32,* 325–338. doi:10.1007/s10979-007-9094-8

McDermott, B. E., Gerbasi, J. B., Quanbeck, C., & Scott, C. L. (2005). Capacity of forensic patients to consent to research: The use of the MacCAT-CR. *Journal of the American Academy of Psychiatry and the Law, 33*(3), 299–307.

McDermott, B. E., Newman, W. J., Meyer, J., Scott, C. L., & Warburton, K. (2017). The utility of an admission screening procedure for patients committed to a state hospital as incompetent to stand trial. *International Journal of Forensic Mental Health, 16*(4), 281–292. doi:http://dx.doi.org/10.1080/14999013.2017.1356890

McDermott, B. E., Quanbeck, C. D., Busse, D., Yastro, K., & Scott, C. L. (2008). The accuracy of risk assessment instruments in the prediction of impulsive versus predatory aggression. *Behavioral Sciences and the Law, 26*(6), 759–777. doi:10.1002/bsl.842

McDermott, B. E., Warburton, K., & Auletta-Young, C. (2019). A longitudinal description of incompetent to stand trial admissions to a state hospital. *CNS Spectrums,* 1–14. doi:10.1017/s1092852919001342

Quanbeck, C. D., McDermott, B. E., Lam, J., Eisenstark, H., Sokolov, G., & Scott, C. L. (2007). Categorization of aggressive acts committed by chronically assaultive state hospital patients. *Psychiatric Services, 58*(4), 521–528. doi:10.1176/ps.2007.58.4.521

Warburton, K., McDermott, B. E., Gale, A., & Stahl, S. M. (2020). A survey of national trends in psychiatric patients found incompetent to stand trial: Reasons for the reinstitutionalization of people with serious mental illness in the United States. *CNS Spectrums, 25*(2), 245–251. doi:10.1017/S1092852919001585

7

Successful Development of Threat Assessment and Management Programming Within a Midwestern University

MARIO J. SCALORA AND ROSA VIÑAS RACIONERO ■

The University of Nebraska-Lincoln has engaged in collaborative behavioral science consultation and training relationships with multiple law enforcement agencies with the goal of developing strategies to prevent targeted violence. This chapter details one such collaborative project: the joint development of a long-standing threat assessment team within a large Midwestern university. This project was modeled after other successful efforts to develop threat assessment and management programming that embedded psychological expertise within law enforcement agencies (see, e.g., Scalora & Zimmerman, 2015).

GENERAL INTRODUCTION TO THREAT ASSESSMENT AND MANAGEMENT

Before describing the development and 10-year program evaluation of threat assessment programing within a Midwestern university, this chapter offers a brief introduction to campus-targeted violence, threat assessment approaches, and the nature of other behavioral health and law enforcement partnerships. Such introductory detail is crucial given that multidisciplinary collaboration regarding threat assessment and management is a relatively recent merging area (Borum, Fein, Vossekuil, & Berglund, 1999; Scalora, Zimmerman, & Wells, 2008).

Campus-targeted violence typically includes a perpetrator posing an identifiable or potentially identifiable threat to an individual, group, or organization prior to an attack (Fein, Vossekuil, & Holden, 1995). Such violence has occurred on college campuses throughout history, affecting students, faculty, and staff across the United States (Drysdale, Modzeleski, & Simons, 2010). For example, attacks at Virginia Tech and Northern Illinois Universities resulted in numerous deaths and nationwide concern about targeted violence (Scalora, Simons, & Van Slyke, 2010).

Although societal attention is often riveted on mass shootings, college campuses are also afflicted by other disruptive and threatening behavior, partner violence, stalking, sexual violence, workplace violence, and extremism activity (Borum, Cornell, Modzeleski, & Jimerson, 2010; Fisher, Cullen, & Turner, 2000; Lauritsen & Reizey, 2013; Roberts, 2005; Spitzberg, 2016). While less destructive than mass casualty violence, these more common forms of interpersonal violence also have the potential to aggravate and evolve into lethal events (e.g., homicide), especially when the problematic individual physically approaches the target.

Given the exceedingly heterogeneous nature and severity of the aforementioned threats, traditional emergency plans for responding to an attack may not suffice to effectively protect an institution and neutralize an attacker before violence ensues (Reddy et al., 2001). Thus, college safety efforts may also focus on preventive rather than solely reactive protection strategies (Modzeleski & Randazzo, 2018). At the core of the prevention strategies lies threat assessment, a behavioral approach that aims to identify and manage individuals at risk for violence (Borum et al., 1999).

Threat assessment typically requires input from multidisciplinary expertise to triage concerning behavior (Fein et al., 2002). Therefore, multidisciplinary teams—also known as threat assessment teams—are considered the gold standard for handling the reports of threats and, subsequently, the management of potentially violent individuals (such management may include, for example, counseling, applying the student code of conduct, and legal restriction of contact between the target and the individual of concern) (Dunkle, Silverstein, & Warmer, 2008). Such teams are currently ubiquitous to collegiate settings (Hollister & Scalora, 2015) and typically encompass a combination of behavioral health, administrative, faculty, and law enforcement personnel. The collaboration of law enforcement and behavioral health is, perhaps, among the most central for the establishment, development, and evaluation of threat assessment teams. Nonetheless, there are still challenges involved in their collaboration.

THE NATURE OF THE COLLABORATION: LAW ENFORCEMENT AND BEHAVIORAL HEALTH PARTNERSHIPS

Behavioral health professionals and law enforcement have a long history of collaborations and partnerships beyond the threat assessment field. For example, psychologists have been involved with law enforcement agencies around issues such as pre-employment selection and fitness-for-duty evaluations (Corey

& Zelig, 2020), hostage negotiations (Butler, Leitenberg, & Fuselier, 1993; DeBernardo, 2004), criminal profiling (Sales, Miller, & Hall, 2005), supporting Special Weapons and Tactical (SWAT) teams (Galyean, Wherry, & Young, 2009), and stress management (Hilgren & Jacobs, 1976).

Co-responding models of collaboration, particularly critical incident teams (CITs) (Augustin & Fagan, 2011) combining law enforcement with embedded behavioral health professionals, are an effort to divert persons with mental illness to mental health resources rather than the criminal justice system. The co-response teams focus on de-escalation strategies as well as diverting mentally ill persons in crisis from arrest and detention to behavioral health care (Kisely et al., 2010; Lamanna et al., 2018; McKenna, Furness, Oakes, & Brown, 2015; Shapiro et al., 2015).

There are several influences promoting such collaboration between law enforcement and behavioral health professionals. One involves well-publicized acts of targeted violence; another is the research highlighting the value of threat assessment as a strategy to assess risk and prevent violent behavior. Whatever the influences, however, there is increasing interest on behalf of public safety agencies in partnerships with behavioral health professionals to develop threat assessment teams.

Behavioral Health Consultation Within Threat Assessment Teams

The partnership between behavioral health and law enforcement in developing threat assessment strategies occurred partially due to the prevalence of mental illnesses—in particular severe mental illness—in individuals at risk of committing acts of targeted violence (Hoffmann, Meloy, Guldimann, & Ermer, 2011; James, Kerrigan, Forfar, Farnham, & Preston, 2010; van der Meer, Bootsma, & Meloy, 2012; Meloy et al., 2004; Pathé et al., 2015; Pathé, Haworth & Lowry, 2016; Scalora, Baumgartner, Zimmerman, et al., 2002; Scalora & Zimmerman, 2015; Sheridan & Pyszora, 2018). From a law enforcement perspective, psychological consultation by mental health professionals is viewed as informing the assessment and management of violence risk (Coggins & Pynchon, 1998; James et al., 2010). Specifically, behavioral health practitioners are better able to evaluate individuals' violence risk and identify those who can be better managed by the mental health system than by the criminal justice system (James, Farnham & Wilson, 2014; Lamb, Weinberger, & DeCuir, 2002). Effective and efficient threat assessment and management therefore necessitate the multidisciplinary collaboration of behavioral health and law enforcement personnel. Mental health knowledge has largely shaped contemporary standards and practices of threat assessment and management (Coggins & Pynchon, 1998; Cornell & Maeng, 2018; James et al., 2014; Pathé et al., 2018; Randazzo & Cameron, 2012; Scalora & Zimmerman, 2015). Accordingly, law enforcement and security organizations have formulated formal threat assessment and management teams based on this mental health–law enforcement collaborative framework in a variety of settings in the United States, United Kingdom (e.g., James et al., 2010, 2014; James & Farnham, 2016), Canada (Randazzo & Cameron, 2012), Australia (e.g., Pathé et al., 2015, 2016, 2018), and the Netherlands (van der Meer et al., 2012).

In the United States, the threat assessment-based mental health–law enforcement collaborative framework appeared linked to efforts aiming at bolstering the protection of public figures (e.g., Coggins & Pynchon, 1998; Phillips, 2008; Scalora, Baumgartner, Callaway, et al., 2002; Scalora & Zimmerman, 2015). Over the past two decades, it has expanded beyond its use exclusively for the protection of public figures and toward more widespread use in workplace settings (Cacialli, 2019; Cornell & Maeng, 2018; Randazzo & Cameron, 2012), primary and secondary schools (e.g., Cornell & Maeng, 2018), and institutions of higher education (e.g., Cacialli, 2019).

The critical role of behavioral health in the threat assessment teams of K-12 schools and institutions of higher education has been widely recognized in the wake of school and campus shootings (e.g., Columbine, Virginia Tech), with teams being mandated by some states (Cacialli, 2019; Cornell & Maeng, 2018). This is largely because a significant proportion of students—in particular university students—who commit targeted violence (e.g., mass school shootings) suffer from a severe mental illness or exhibit symptoms indicative of a severe mental illness (Newman & Fox, 2009; see Cacialli, 2019, for a review). In addition to severe mental illness, additional challenges for mental health practice appear when evaluating and managing violence risk within higher education settings (Cacialli, 2019), including appropriate consideration of the mental, social, cognitive, and moral development of the student and the legal and ethical dilemmas related to client–patient confidentiality, mandatory reporting, and dual relationships.

Although partnerships between law enforcement and behavioral health have been successful in a variety of contexts, such partnerships must be developed with an awareness of the inherent challenges.

Challenges in Consulting with Law Enforcement Agencies

There are substantial challenges in consulting with public safety organizations given the nature of organizational structure and dynamics that affect how consultants can gain trust and credibility within the organization (Scalora, 2009). For this reason, to be effective, behavioral health consultants must be aware of the nature of law enforcement activity. For example, law enforcement professionals are often exposed to emotionally demanding interpersonal situations, including illness, violence, and death (Bakker & Heuven, 2006). Law enforcement officers may sometimes deal with unanticipated situations involving safety implications. Such situations demand real-time decisive action requiring discretion that must be practiced within broadly defined protocols. Officers must make assessments during sometimes ambiguous situations that may make information-gathering difficult—especially during hostile and combative situations. The assessment and intervention activities generally occur within a team structure, requiring coordination within real time. As Devine (2002) noted, every situation encountered may provide unique circumstances, which often means that responses must be crafted "on the fly," using the professional's discretion. The team structure within law enforcement agencies utilizes a hierarchical framework that oversees command and control functions (Klimoski & Jones, 1995). This hierarchical framework contains a chain of command that must be respected by both insiders and outsiders. Disagreements with command decisions must occur formally within the chain of command. Any informal challenges to such decision-making, especially from consultants, must take place in a discrete manner.

Law enforcement professionals' decision-making and the resulting outcomes may come under scrutiny both inside and outside of the organization from a range of constituencies served. Many public safety professionals are in positions involving high public visibility and high organizational scrutiny. Furthermore, negative outcomes are often publicly displayed through increased external inquiry. Finally, as in many high-risk professions, training for law enforcement and other public safety professionals often involves strong mentorship. On-the-job learning is typically action- and procedure-driven.

The Development of a Threat Assessment Team at a Midwestern University

A proficient knowledge of threat assessment is necessary but not sufficient when developing a threat assessment team. Adequate consultation skills and partnership experience with law enforcement are as important as technical knowledge. This section offers a detailed account of how the first author assisted and coordinated with law enforcement to develop a threat assessment team. We offer details highlighting the efforts to ensure effectiveness and adherence to threat assessment principles over the 10-year period of this team's development and implementation.

The development of threat assessment strategies could not happen without the buy-in and joint ownership of University law enforcement and administrative leadership. In addition, both University law enforcement and administrative leadership agreed that threat assessment activity would be overseen by the Chief of University Police, given the key safety responsibilities entailed. While such recognition of law enforcement leadership was consistent with public safety planning, it was also critical to ensure that the threat assessment process would not be perceived as heavy-handed or punitive in nature—and to support the values consistent with a university campus environment. This was highlighted both as policy was developed and during engagement with various stakeholders: threat assessment would de-escalate conflict and use interventions that promote dignity and respect. Such threat assessment was portrayed as preventive rather than reactive, with the goal of promoting an open and safe campus environment. Policy development reflected such values.

While receiving the buy-in and approval from key administrative stakeholders, the consultants and law enforcement leadership drew heavily on the relevant threat assessment literature (e.g., Deisinger, Randazzo, O'Neill, & Savage, 2008) to develop the structure of the campus threat assessment partnership and the roles of threat assessment team members. The consultants analyzed cases of targeted violence already being managed by University Police. The results indicated that the University was experiencing concerning behavior from an array of internal sources (students, staff, and faculty) as well as from a sizeable number of individuals not affiliated with the University. As a result, the threat assessment partnership was structured to address an array of potential threats to campus safety, not just those related to students of concern. Furthermore, to alleviate concerns regarding civil liberties as well as to remain consistent with threat assessment principles (e.g., Deisinger, Randazzo, O'Neill, & Savage, 2008; Fein et al., 2002), it was critical to highlight that the triggering conditions and subsequent assessment process would be behavior- not profile-based. As a result, the campus threat assessment strategy was framed to focus on "troubling behavior as opposed to troubled persons." Troubling behaviors were identified as any behavior directed toward campus stakeholders or the campus in general as potentially

- Causing harm or potential to cause harm, or
- Threatening to life safety, or
- Potentially causing serious damage to University property or operations.

The threat assessment team was designed to incorporate flexibility regarding the nature of the concerning behavior presented. The core of the threat assessment team included police personnel and psychological consultants with training in threat assessment. The police members also needed experience in conducting investigations and gathering background information.

Additional team members would assist as needed, including

- University administration
- Faculty
- Legal counsel
- Human resources
- Student/Judicial affairs
- Campus mental health services
- Campus employee assistance programs

The specific members of the Threat Assessment Team comprised campus personnel who have decision-making skills in dealing with troubling situations. The team's primary focus was to facilitate communication and coordination when aware of a safety issue and to coordinate resources to address cases involving lower concern for violence. The larger team reviewed specific cases to ensure appropriate services and interventions and to suggest procedural changes for the future.

The psychological consultants served several roles in the development and functioning of the team, including

- Assisting University Chief of Police with *developing* the structure of the team and meeting with various stakeholders to detail the nature of the university threat assessment team. Such meetings were focused on alleviating concerns related to the team's role relative to other university administrative functions. In addition, efforts were made to note how safeguards concerning confidentiality and privacy of various parties would be maintained. Confidentiality protocols were developed because information could be drawn from confidential sources. Case-specific issues and information were treated as confidential to protect privacy and civil rights.
- Providing periodic *training* to University Police and members of the Threat Assessment Team. Training of university police was multifaceted and focused on threat assessment risk factors and management strategies. The consultants also provided training on issues of mental health and the mental health system (e.g., nature of mental illness, interviewing persons with mental illness, nature of mental health and risk assessment principles).
- Providing *case consultation*; as an integrated team member, and at the discretion of the police investigator agent, consultants assisted with the determination of risk and the development of management strategies. Consultation was generally geared toward determining whether an individual is likely to engage in concerning behavior or to provide insight on case management concerns.
- The consultants also served in a *liaison* role with the mental health community. The behavioral health consultants worked to enhance the familiarity of the mental health community with the nature of the threat assessment team and helped develop collaborative relationships in cases in which persons of interest were involved with both systems. Specific engagement might address issues regarding the exchange of information and duty to warn/protect issues when applicable.
- The consultants, with the assistance of graduate students and other trainees, assisted with *program evaluation and research* activity relevant to threat assessment team activity as case outcome. Commentators (Randazzo & Cameron, 2012; Scalora & Zimmerman, 2015) emphasize the importance of utilizing the research expertise of mental health professionals to further improve the effectiveness of threat assessment and management practices. More specifically, knowledgeable mental health professionals should conduct research to investigate trends in violent behavior and threatening activity; identify underlying motivations, mechanisms, and risk factors associated with such behavior; and evaluate the outcomes of threat assessment and management teams.

A 10-Year Evaluation of the Midwestern Threat Assessment Team

To evaluate the impact of the threat assessment team's activity as well as its adherence to relevant processes, the consultants reviewed records of 322 threat assessment cases reported to the University Police between 2006 and 2016 (Viñas-Racionero, 2018). Overall, the threat assessment practices of this team were oriented toward managing risk while simultaneously enabling the person of concern to continue his or her education at (or remain affiliated with) the University, provided that the individual did not pose a considerable risk to others, which is consistent with the principles of threat management (Cacialli, 2019; Cornell & Maeng, 2018). In other words, school and campus threat assessment were concerned not only with public safety, but also with the educational needs of the person of concern. The main findings of this program evaluation are summarized here.

Finding 1: There is no single profile of a problematic individual. There was no readily identifiable single profile of an individual engaging in concerning activity, as has been reported by others (e.g., Burns, Dean, & Jacob-Timm, 2001; Borum, Fein, & Vossekuil, 2012; Fein & Vossekuil, 1999; Gill, 2015; Horgan, 2008; Monahan, 2012; O'Toole, 2000). This initial finding underscores that the focus of the threat assessment team's investigative activity should be the individual's discrete behaviors and not their characteristics or group membership.

Furthermore, such concerning individuals typically had disparate levels of involvement within the educational setting. Most of them were affiliated with the university (about 76% were students, faculty, or staff), while the remaining individuals were not directly university-affiliated. This result is not surprising given the wide-ranging nature and activities of college institutions, which might attract individuals who are not directly affiliated to the campus (e.g., athletic events). This spoke to the continuing need for the threat assessment team to address and screen multiple sources of concerning behavior—not just focusing on specific sources of concerning behavior from within the university.

Finding 2: Individuals who engaged in concerning behavior often presented with mental health problems. According to the results of the program evaluation study, half of the persons of concern presented with psychological problems that varied in severity and type. About half exhibited active symptoms of severe mental health disorder (e.g., hallucinatory disturbances, delusional ideation, thought disorganization). Between 10% and 20% also had a history of suicidality (18%) or homicidality (12%) as well as a history of alcohol (19%) or substance abuse (19%). A nuanced analysis of these individuals' behavior suggested that acute symptoms of severe mental disorder appeared to be foundational for escalating the risk for repeated communications, physical approach, and targeted violence, consistent with severe mental illness as a risk factor for targeted violence (Marquez & Scalora, 2011; Scalora, Washington, Casady, & Newell, 2003).

Individuals who experienced delusions or hallucinations displayed rigid beliefs that often led to very personal and inaccurate perceptions of their reality (i.e., personal grievances that were delusional in nature). For such individuals, these beliefs often seemed to justify their actions and were conveyed using intense communications designed to publicize their cause against the target and other third parties. These individuals often felt entitled to behave as they did and could not understand others questioning their reasons, which could be persecutory and conspiracy-based. Therefore, they were more likely to persist in their behavior.

Finding 3: The majority of threat situations stemmed from a grievance against the target. Most threatening behavior stemmed from unresolved long-standing conflicts or grievances between individuals who knew each other (as in 80% of these 322 cases). Threat assessment investigations often commenced when receiving reports of such concerns after conflicts escalated. Such escalated conflicts mostly involved threats to harm others or behaviors that indicated a capability or intent to engage in violence (e.g., physical assaults, angry outbursts, stalking behavior, attack preparatory behaviors). This finding highlighted the need to consider the history of conflict between the person of concern and the target during the assessment phase.

Finding 4: The majority of cases tended to involve multiple targets. One of the most relevant findings of this study is that threatening situations often involved substantial target dispersion—the dissemination of grievance or concerning behavior among multiple targets. For example, 200 of 322 cases involved multiple targets, and 122 of 322 cases focused mainly on a specific individual. Such targets may or may not have been preemptively identified by the individual of concern. This finding underscored the importance of continuing to gather information after the initial report so additional targets are not overlooked.

A closer analysis of the data suggested that target dispersion is a widely varying dynamic. It emerged in different situations, with different type of actors, and across different durations. First, target dispersion was seen when individuals leaked their violent ideation to others (i.e., expressed violent intentions to third parties via statements or social media), which has also been described in other studies of school violence (Hoffmann et al., 2011; Reddy et al., 2001). In this regard, target dispersion entails "expanding the audience" of the grievance.

Finding 5: Individuals of concern detailed personal grievances. Another notable finding was the identification of a broad range of motives that were communicated during problematic activity. In accordance with prior findings on harassment activity (Borum, 2014; Scalora et al., 2002), most of the motivations for concerning behavior were personal in nature (65% of the cases). Specifically, data suggested that individuals of concern had difficulty coping with personal failures, losses (e.g., an intimate relationship), or individual stressors (particularly academic, work, or legal issues) and communicated their concerns via requests for help or emotional statements indicating that they felt undermined or unsafe. As observed in other types of harassment activity (Marquez & Scalora, 2011), the 2006–2016 threat management study suggested that the more personal the grievance, the more persistent the problematic behavior became. In addition, if the underlying personal motives and emotions were not resolved, motivations such as retaliation and intimidation were likely to appear in the grievances communication themes.

In these situations, the targets were likely to feel unsafe, which triggered their reporting of problematic behavior to law enforcement.

Finding 6: Cases reported tended to involve high-intensity effort. Over the 10-year span of cases, the problematic activity observed on the college campus spanned multiple contacts over an extended period of time. On average, the targets were contacted 11 times via multiple communication channels at different locations, both on and off campus, over a period of 6 months. Most contacts consisted of a combination of face-to-face threatening interactions (approximately 55%), emails and posts online (45.2%), and phone calls (24.4%) in which the individuals expressed their grievances or anger. In approximately 75% of the cases, the individuals articulated some form of violent intent (e.g., direct, conditional, or vague threats). A minority of the cases included instances of physical or sexual violence, interest in or use of weapons, or self-harming behavior (15%). Most of these instances of violent behavior occurred before the university police became involved in the threat assessment case. For example, 67% of cases involving physical violence stemmed from partner violence that spilled into the academic environment.

Finding 7: Multiple threat assessment interventions were needed to address concerning situations. Concerning behaviors were not always reported in a timely manner. Overall, the threat assessment process started after the targets perceived that their safety was at risk. Given that targets often vacillate in their perception of risk, their threshold for reporting problematic activity might vary as well (see Hollister, Scalora, Hoff, & Marquez, 2014). Accordingly, only one-fourth of the cases were opened within 24 hours of the *first* incident of problematic activity (28%). The majority of the targets sought the help of either law enforcement or the threat assessment team directly after escalation of a long-standing, unresolved conflict with the problematic individual (57%). Thus, the data highlighted that investigators and threat assessment team members should anticipate that initial reports of threat situation are an incomplete representation of the threatening situation.

Simultaneous interventions were often necessary. Threat assessment investigations might expand several years. Specifically, cases lasted 1 year on average (range from 1 day to 9 years) and were addressed through several interventions. Virtually all cases needed different information-gathering strategies (93%) and required restrictive subject-focused plans, target safety plans, or both types of direct interventions (98%). These results seem logical in light of the severity of the cases (e.g., threatening face-to-face interactions, physical and sexual violence, and violent ideation). The implementation of these management strategies was dynamic, flexible, and fluid, depending on the behavior of the individuals of concern as well as the targets' vulnerability. To decide the appropriate level of intervention, an effective triage of cases was necessary.

Cases were triaged and a determination made of the imminence of potential violence. Consistent with scientific literature, the threat management process often started by assessing any signs of imminent violence or in reaction to a violent event (Bondü & Scheithauer, 2014; Harrell, 2013; Meloy et al., 2011; Meloy,

Hoffmann, Roshdi, & Guldimann, 2014; Scalora, Baugartner, Zimmerman, et al., 2002). Approximately 20% of cases were opened for concerns related to current violence or homicidal ideation, which triggered an immediate response from law enforcement. Such immediate responses included legal actions (e.g., arrest), academic sanctions, mandatory mental health treatment, or some combination of these.

When the risk of violence was not deemed imminent, investigators started the threat management process by assessing and monitoring problematic activity. Specifically, investigators within threat assessment teams gathered as much information as possible to determine the seriousness of the threat and the veracity of the facts reported to them (e.g., motivation, intention to approach or attack the target, determination of individuals' mental condition, analysis of consistency between communications and behavior, etc.) (93% of cases), which is consistent with typical threat assessment practices (see Randazzo & Plummer, 2009; Reddy et al., 2001).

Assessment and information-gathering were crucial. Half of the cases studied required direct interviews with the individuals of concern and the targets. Between 30% and 40% of the cases required consulting and gathering information with university resources such as student affairs or mental health services. Another 40% of the cases involved coordination and information sharing with community entities such as other law enforcement agencies, district attorney's office, private corporations, or other community resources (e.g., social service agencies, medical and behavioral health practitioners). Basically, the focus of the assessment phase was to determine whether the individual had a genuine intent to harm the target.

Restrictive interventions were used when other alternatives failed. Depending on the person of concern's appraised risk for harming the target, the information-gathering strategies were combined with interventions that required the problematic individual to cease contact with the target(s). As recommended in the scientific literature (Scalora et al., 2008), these interventions were also designed to redirect these individuals to services that would mitigate their grievances. Furthermore, individuals of concern might be required to attend psychological treatment to address different mental health concerns that could be exacerbating their behavior (e.g., hallucinatory experiences, delusional ideation, severe agitation, homicidality, suicidality, or substance use) (26% of cases in the study) (Farkas & Tsukayama, 2012; MacKenzie & James, 2011). If not engaged in treatment voluntarily, such treatment may be leveraged through student or employee disciplinary standards or, in some limited cases, judicial requirements. If these less intense interventions did not suffice, threat assessment professionals resorted to interventions that prevented problematic individuals from approaching the targets, such as severe academic sanctions (16% of cases ended up in a suspension or expulsion) or legal sanctions (16% involved arrest, 14% involved barring from campus, 17% involved citations for charges such as terroristic threat or harassment).

Consultation played a crucial role in successful intervention. Consistent with the literature (e.g., Deisinger et al., 2008), the role of the threat assessment team varied depending on case characteristics. The data indicate that the threat assessment team was mostly utilized for consultation purposes. Team members other than law enforcement officers were engaged directly in a case as part of the threat management strategy (e.g., student affairs meeting weekly with students of concern to monitor their progress). The results suggest that the threat assessment team was generally effective in tailoring interventions and management strategies to the level of risk posed by the concerning behavior.

Lessons Learned

Reflection on the nature of the consultation and the available data from the 10-year program evaluation suggested several lessons learned from this partnership between behavioral health and law enforcement. Behavioral health consultants must recognize the need to be "good team players" who recognize that their role as an integrated team member or consultant differs from their role and authority in the clinical setting (Augustin & Fagan, 2011).

A key lesson learned was the frequent need for continuous training at a level not initially anticipated. This collaborative behavioral health–law enforcement partnership requires periodic attention to training to ensure adherence to principles, reliability of process, and continuity of practice, which are typically best assessed thorough a formalized program evaluation such as the one described in this chapter. Given frequent turnover (e.g., promotions and changes in duty) for law enforcement and other team personnel, periodic training in mental health and threat assessment issues is critical to ensure continuity of processes. Training and follow-up consultation must focus on adherence to relevant threat assessment and risk assessment principles. Reliability as well as adherence to process can often degrade over the time following training if supervision or follow-up checks do not occur. Furthermore, follow-up consultation and data collection processes must focus on ensuring adherence to community policing and related values to avoid reliance on punitive or heavy-handed approaches.

A pervasive challenge is the need to constantly engage and educate the various campus and community stakeholders of the nature and benefits of the threat assessment process. Higher educational institutions, by their nature, tend to have significant turnover of students, administrators, and faculty. Such turnover necessitates frequent outreach and education regarding safety procedures as well as the nature of the threat assessment process. The level of such constant outreach was unexpected and can sometimes be rather demanding in addition to implementing the threat assessment and management programming.

Particularly challenging is when campuses are beset by controversial situations that tax safety resources—including threat assessment efforts. For example, campuses often encounter controversial events (e.g., controversial speaker, protests) which may sometimes escalate into multiple threatening communications directed toward campus personnel and the institution. These events tax the resources of campus law enforcement and the threat assessment team. In the case of controversial events, different parties may question whether threatening communications even existed—requiring even more education concerning the role of the threat assessment team.

Behavioral health consultants must be mindful of potential ethical dilemmas and other challenges. Dietz and Reese (1986) highlighted common dilemmas faced by mental health professionals working on behalf of law enforcement agencies relating to conflicts in value and norms as well as the erosion of professional identity. Because of different backgrounds, there may be differences in values and norms held by law enforcement professionals and mental health professionals that could lead to conflict if not addressed. Dietz and Reese (1986) suggest that mental health consultants recognize such differences and direct communications to the appropriate level within the command hierarchy. Consultants must also be mindful, given the sensitivity of threat assessment cases, to obtain the permission of those in authority before speaking with the media or publishing any identifiable information about cases or agency activities. In addition, mental health professionals working must be sensitive to their law enforcement colleagues' concerns and needs; mental health professionals need to "stay in their lane" to avoid engaging in activity better suited for law enforcement (e.g., determining when arrest is necessary, overidentification with law enforcement role).

Consultants must be constantly aware of the potential for multiple roles within this public safety context. Threat assessment activity by the behavioral health consultant often involves indirect assessment of the behavior of concern. Significant ethical issues may arise when indirect assessment—methods that do not involve face-to-face interaction—is conducted (Acklin, 2018). Indirect behavioral methods are commonly utilized in clinical, forensic, law enforcement, public safety, and national security settings. Given the nature of such consultation, tensions may emerge between the principles of beneficence and duty to society. In this chapter, we have discussed the use of indirect approaches to personality assessment and some ethical ramifications. The consultant must remain aware of the potential for harm to the various parties concerned. Furthermore, consultants must constantly be mindful of the limitations of their opinions and constantly assert such limitations with their colleagues during deliberations. Overconfidence in such opinions may be particularly concerning during indirect assessment contexts given the limitation of information available and dynamic nature of risk.

REFERENCES

Acklin, M. W. (2018). Beyond the boundaries: Ethical issues in the practice of indirect personality assessment in non-health service psychology. *Journal of Personality Assessment, 102*(2), 269–277.

Augustin, D., & Fagan, T. J. (2011). Roles for mental health professionals in critical law enforcement incidents: An overview. *Psychological Services, 8,* 166–177. doi:10.1037/a0024104.

Bakker, A., & Heuven, E. (2006). Emotional dissonance, burnout, and in-role performance among nurses and police officers. *International Journal of Stress Management,*
13, 423–440.

Bondü, R., & Scheithauer, H. (2014). Leaking and death-threats by students: A study
in German schools. *School Psychology International, 35*, 592–608. doi:10.1177/
0143034314552346

Borum, R. (2014). Psychological vulnerabilities and propensities for involvement
in violent extremism. *Behavioral Sciences & the Law, 32*, 286–305. doi:10.1002/
bsl.2110

Borum, R., Cornell, D. G., Modzeleski, W., & Jimerson, S. R. (2010). What can be done
about school shootings? A review of the evidence. *Educational Researcher, 39*, 27–
37. doi:10.3102/0013189X09357620

Borum, R., Fein, R., & Vossekuil, B. (2012). A dimensional approach to analyzing lone
offender terrorism. *Aggression and Violent Behavior, 17*, 389–396. doi:10.1016/
j.avb.2012.04.003

Borum, R., Fein, R., Vossekuil, B., & Berglund, J. (1999). Threat assessment: Defining
an approach for evaluating risk of targeted violence. *Behavioral Sciences & the Law,*
17, 323–337.

Burns, M. K., Dean, V. J., & Jacob-Timm, S. (2001). Assessment of violence potential
among school children: Beyond profiling. *Psychology in the Schools, 38*, 239–247.
doi:10.1002/pits.1014

Butler, W. M., Leitenberg, H., & Fuselier, G. D. (1993). The use of mental health professional consultants to police hostage negotiation teams. *Behavioral Sciences & the
Law, 11*, 213–221.

Cacialli, D. O. (2019). The unique role and special considerations of mental health
professionals on threat assessment teams at institutions of higher education.
International Journal of Law and Psychiatry, 62, 32–44.

Coggins, M. H., & Pynchon, M. R. (1998). Mental health consultation to law enforcement: Secret Service development of a mental health liaison program. *Behavioral
Sciences & the Law, 16*, 407–422.

Corey, D., & Zelig, M. (2020). *Evaluations of police suitability and fitness for duty.*
New York: Oxford University Press.

Cornell, D., & Maeng, J. (2018). Statewide implementation of threat assessment in
Virginia K-12 schools. *Contemporary School Psychology, 22*, 116–124.

DeBernardo, C. R. (2004). The psychologist's role in hostage negotiations. *International
Journal of Emergency Mental Health, 6*, 39–42.

Dietz, P. E., & Reese, J. T. (1986). The perils of police psychology: 10 strategies for
minimizing role conflicts when providing mental health services and consultation
to law enforcement agencies. *Behavioral Sciences & the Law, 4*, 385–400.

Deisinger, G., Randazzo, M., O'Neill, D., & Savage, J. (2008). *The handbook for campus
threat assessment and management teams.* Boston, Massachusetts: Applied Risk
Management.

Devine, D. J. (2002). A review and integration of classification systems relevant to teams
in organizations. *Group Dynamics: Theory, Research, and Practice, 6*, 291–310.

Drysdale, D. A., Modzeleski, W., & Simons, A. B. (2010). *Campus attacks: Targeted violence affecting institutions of higher education.* Washington, DC: US Secret Service,
US Department of Homeland Security, Office of Safe and Drug-Free Schools, US

Department of Education, and Federal Bureau of Investigation, US Department of Justice.

Dunkle, J., Silverstein, Z., & Warner, S. (2008). Managing violent and other troubling students: The role of threat assessment on campus. *Journal of College and University Law, 34*(3), 585–635.

Farkas, G. M., & Tsukayama, J. K. (2012). An integrative approach to threat assessment and management: Security and mental health response to a threatening client. *Work: Journal of Prevention, Assessment & Rehabilitation, 42*, 9–14.

Fein, R. A., & Vossekuil, B. (1999). Assassination in the United States: An operational study of recent assassins, attackers, and near-lethal approachers. *Journal of Forensic Sciences, 44*, 321–333.

Fein, R. A., Vossekuil, B., & Holden, G. A. (1995). *Threat assessment: An approach to prevent targeted violence* (*Vol. 2*). Washington, DC: US Department of Justice, Office of Justice Programs, National Institute of Justice.

Fein, R., Vossekuil, B., Pollack, W., Borum, R., Modzeleski, W., & Reddy, M. (2002). *Threat assessment in schools: A guide to managing threatening situations and to creating safe school climates*. Washington, DC: US Secret Service and US Department of Education.

Fisher, B. S., Cullen, F. T., & Turner, M. G. (2000). *The sexual victimization of college women* (NCJRS Publication No. 182369). Washington, DC: US Department of Justice, National Criminal Justice Reference Service.

Galyean, K. D., Wherry, J. N., & Young, A. T. (2009). Valuation of services offered by mental health professionals in SWAT team members: A study of the Lubbock, Texas SWAT team. *Journal of Police and Criminal Psychology, 24*, 51–58.

Gill, P. (2015). Toward a scientific approach to identifying and understanding indicators of radicalization and terrorist intent: Eight key problems. *Journal of Threat Assessment and Management, 2*, 187–191. doi:2169-4842/15

Harrell, E. (2013, April). *Workplace violence against government employees, 1994–2011.* (NCJ Publication No. 242349). Washington, DC: US Department of Justice, Office of Justice Programs. Bureau of Justice Statistics.

Hilgren, J., & Jacobs, P. (1976). The consulting psychologist's emerging role in law enforcement. *Professional Psychology, 7*, 256–266.

Hoffmann, J., Meloy, J. R., Guldimann, A., & Ermer, A. (2011). Attacks on German public figures, 1968–2004: Warning behaviors, potentially lethal and non-lethal acts, psychiatric status, and motivations. *Behavioral Sciences & the Law, 29*, 155–179. doi:10.1002/bsl.979

Hollister, B. A., & Scalora, M. J. (2015). Broadening campus threat assessment beyond mass shootings. *Aggression and Violent Behavior, 25*(Part A), 43–53. doi:10.1016/j.avb.2015.07.005

Hollister, B., Scalora, M., Hoff, S., & Marquez, A. (2014). Exposure to preincident behavior and reporting in college students. *Journal of Threat Assessment and Management, 1*, 129–143. doi:10.1037/tam0000015

Horgan, J. H. (2008). From profiles to pathways and roots to routes: Perspectives from psychology on radicalization into terrorism. *Annals of the American Academy of Political and Social Science, 618*, 80–94. doi:10.1177/0002716208317539

James, D. V., & Farnham, F. R. (2016). Outcome and efficacy of interventions by a public figure threat assessment and management unit: A mirrored study of concerning behaviors and police contacts before and after intervention. *Behavioral Sciences & the Law, 34,* 660–680.

James, D. V., Farnham, F. R., & Wilson, S. P. (2014). The Fixated Threat Assessment Centre: Implementing a joint police and psychiatric approach to risk assessment and management in public figure threat cases. In J. R. Meloy & J. Hoffman (Eds.), *International handbook of threat assessment* (pp. 299–320). New York: Oxford University Press.

James, D. V., Kerrigan, T. R., Forfar, R., Farnham, F. R., & Preston, L. F. (2010). The Fixated Threat Assessment Centre: Preventing harm and facilitating care. *The Journal of Forensic Psychiatry & Psychology, 21,* 521–536.

James, D. V., Meloy, J. R., Mullen, P. E., Pathé, M. T., Farnham, F. R., Preston, L. F., & Darnley, B. J. (2010). Abnormal attentions toward the British Royal Family: Factors associated with approach and escalation. *Journal of the American Academy of Psychiatry and the Law, 38,* 329–340.

Kisely, S., Campbell, L. A., Peddle, S., Hare, S., Pyche, M., Spicer, D., & Moore, B. (2010). A controlled before-and-after evaluation of a mobile crisis partnership between mental health and police services in Nova Scotia. *Canadian Journal of Psychiatry, 55,* 662–668.

Klimoski, R., & Jones, R. G. (1995). Staffing for effective group decision making: Key issues in matching people and teams. In R. Guzzo, E. Salas, & Associates (Eds.), *Team effectiveness and decision making in organizations* (pp. 291–332). San Francisco: Jossey-Bass.

Lamanna, D., Shapiro, G. K., Kirst, M., Matheson, F. I., Nakhost, A., & Stergiopoulos, V. (2018). Co-responding police–mental health programmes: Service user experiences and outcomes in a large urban centre. *International Journal of Mental Health Nursing, 27,* 891–900.

Lamb, H. R., Weinberger, L. E., & DeCuir Jr., W. J. (2002). The police and mental health. *Psychiatric Services, 53,* 1266–1271.

Lauritsen, J. L., & Rezey, M. L. (2013, September). *Measuring the prevalence of crime with the National Crime Victimization Survey.* (NCJ Publication No. 241656). Washington, DC: US Department of Justice, National Criminal Justice Reference Service.

MacKenzie, R. D., & James, D. V. (2011). Management and treatment of stalkers: Problems, options, and solutions. *Behavioral Sciences & the Law, 29,* 220–239. doi:10.1002/bsl.980

Marquez, A., & Scalora, M. J. (2011). Problematic approach of legislators: Differentiating stalking from isolated incidents. *Criminal Justice and Behavior, 38,* 1115–1126. doi:10.1177/0093854811420847

McKenna, B., Furness, T., Oakes, J., & Brown, S. (2015). Police and mental health clinician partnership in response to mental health crisis: A qualitative study. *International Journal of Mental Health Nursing, 24,* 386–393.

Meloy, J. R., Hoffmann, J., Roshdi, K., & Guldimann, A. (2014). Some warning behaviors discriminate between school shooters and other students of concern. *Journal of Threat Assessment and Management, 1,* 203–211. doi:10.1037/tam0000020

Meloy, J., James, D., Farnham, F., Mullen, P., Pathé, M., Darnley, B., & Preston, L. (2004). A research review of public figure threats, approaches, attacks, and assassinations in the United States. *Journal of Forensic Sciences, 49,* 1–8.

Meloy, J. R., James, D. V., Mullen, P. E., Pathé, M. T., Farnham, F. R., Preston, L. F., & Darnley, B. J. (2011). Factors associated with escalation and problematic approaches toward public figures. *Journal of Forensic Sciences, 56*(Suppl. 1), S128–S135. doi:10.1111/j.1556-4029.2010.01574.x

Modzeleski, W., & Randazzo, M. R. (2018). School threat assessment in the USA: Lessons learned from 15 years of teaching and using the federal 'l to prevent school shootings. *Contemporary School Psychology, 22*, 109–115. doi:10.1007/s40688-018-0188-8

Monahan, J. (2012). The individual risk assessment of terrorism. *Psychology, Public Policy, and Law, 18*, 167–205. http://dx.doi.org/10.1037/a0025792

Newman, K., & Fox, C. (2009). Rampage shootings in American high school and college settings, 2002–2008. *American Behavioral Scientist, 52*, 1286–1308.

O'Toole, M. E. (2000). *The school shooter: A threat assessment perspective.* Washington, DC: US Department of Justice, Federal Bureau of Investigation

Pathé, M. T., Haworth, D. J., Goodwin, T. A., Holman, A. G., Amos, S. J., Winterbourne, P., & Day, L. (2018). Establishing a joint agency response to the threat of lone-actor grievance-fuelled violence. *Journal of Forensic Psychiatry & Psychology, 29*, 37–52.

Pathé, M. T., Haworth, D. J., & Lowry, T. J. (2016). Mitigating the risk posed by fixated persons at major events: A joint police-mental health intelligence approach. *Journal of Policing, Intelligence and Counter Terrorism, 11*, 63–72.

Pathé, M. T., Lowry, T., Haworth, D. J., Webster, D. M., Mulder, M. J., Winterbourne, P., & Briggs, C. J. (2015). Assessing and managing the threat posed by fixated persons in Australia. *Journal of Forensic Psychiatry & Psychology, 26*, 425–438.

Phillips, R. T. M. (2008). Preventing assassination: Psychiatric consultation to the United States Secret Service. In J. R. Meloy, L. Sheridan, & J. Hoffman (Eds.), *Stalking, threatening, and attacking public figures: A psychological and behavioral analysis* (pp. 363–385). New York: Oxford University Press.

Randazzo, M. R., & Cameron, J. K. (2012). From presidential protection to campus security: A brief history of threat assessment in North American schools and colleges. *Journal of College Student Psychotherapy, 26*, 277–290.

Randazzo, M. R., & Plummer, E. (2009, November). *Implementing behavioral threat assessment on campus. A Virginia Tech demonstration project.* Blacksburg, VA: Virginia Polytechnic Institute and State University. https://www.threatassessment.vt.edu/Implementing_Behavioral_Threat_Assessment.pdf

Reddy, M., Borum, R., Berglund, J., Vossekuil, B., Fein, R., & Modzeleski, W. (2001). Evaluating risk for targeted violence in schools: Comparing risk assessment, threat assessment, and other approaches. *Psychology in the Schools, 38*, 157–172.

Roberts, K. A. (2005). Associated characteristics of stalking following the termination of romantic relationships. *Applied Psychology in Criminal Justice, 1*, 15–35.

Sales, B. D., Miller, M. O., & Hall, S. R. (2005). Law enforcement. In B. D. Sales, M. O. Miller, & S. R. Hall (Eds.), *Laws affecting clinical practice* (pp.153–155). Washington, DC: American Psychological Association.

Scalora, M. J. (2009). Top down and bottom up: Consulting within hierarchical organizations. In K. F. Hays (Ed.), *Performance psychology in action.* Washington DC: American Psychological Association.

Scalora, M. J., Baumgartner, J. V., Callaway, D., Zimmerman, W., Hatch-Maillette, M. A., Covell, C. N., . . . Washington, D. O. (2002). An epidemiological assessment of problematic contacts to members of Congress. *Journal of Forensic Sciences, 47*, 1360–1364.

Scalora, M. J., Baumgartner, J. V., Zimmerman, W., Callaway, D., Hatch-Maillette, M., Covell, C., . . . Washington, D. (2002). Risk factors for approach behavior toward the US Congress. *Journal of Threat Assessment, 2*, 35–55. http://dx.doi.org/ 10.1300/ J177v02n02_03

Scalora, M. J., Simons, A., & Van Slyke. S. (2010). Campus safety: Assessing and managing threats. *FBI Law Enforcement Bulletin, 79, 1–10.*

Scalora, M. J., Washington, D. O., Casady, T., & Newell, S. P. (2003). Nonfatal workplace violence risk factors: Data from a police contact sample. *Journal of Interpersonal Violence, 18*, 310–327. doi:10.1177/0886260502250092

Scalora, M. J., & Zimmerman, W. (2015). Then and now: Tracking a federal agency's threat assessment activity through two decades with an eye toward the future. *Journal of Threat Assessment and Management, 2*, 268–274.

Scalora, M. J., Zimmerman, W., & Wells, D. G. (2008). Use of threat assessment for the protection of Congress. In J. R. Meloy, L. Sheridan, & J. Hoffmann (Eds.)., *Stalking, threats, and attacks against public figures* (pp. 425–434). New York: Oxford University Press.

Sheridan, L., & Pyszora, N. (2018). Fixations on the police: An exploratory analysis. *Journal of Threat Assessment and Management, 5*(2), 63–74.

Shapiro, G. K., Cusi, A., Kirst, M., O'Campo, P., Nakhost, A., & Stergiopoulos, V. (2015). Co-responding police-mental health programs: A review. *Administration and Policy in Mental Health and Mental Health Services Research, 42*, 606–620.

Spitzberg, B. H. (2016). Acknowledgment of unwanted pursuit, threats, assault, and stalking in a college population. *Psychology of Violence.* Advanced online publication. doi:10.1037/a0040205

van der Meer, B. B., Bootsma, B., & Meloy, J. R. (2012). Disturbing communications and problematic approaches to the Dutch Royal Family. *Journal of Forensic Psychiatry & Psychology, 23*, 571–589.

Viñas-Racionero, R. (2018). *A multifactorial model of threat assessment activity applied to educational settings* (Doctoral dissertation). University of Nebraska-Lincoln, Lincoln.

8

Using an Academic–Practice Partnership to Develop and Implement an Empirically Informed Approach to Juvenile Probation Case Management in Philadelphia

NAOMI E. GOLDSTEIN, JEANNE MCPHEE,
ELIZABETH GALE-BENTZ, AND RENA KREIMER* ∎

Every year, hundreds of thousands of youth are ordered to participate in community-based probation supervision, either through formal disposition or as a form of informal or voluntary probation prior to or in lieu of adjudication (Hockenberry & Puzzanchera, 2018). In many jurisdictions throughout the United States, juvenile probation policies and practices reflect the structure of adult probation in many ways—probation officers closely monitor youth behavior and expect full compliance with court-ordered conditions. Despite their efforts, many youth are unable to adhere to the numerous probation requirements imposed on them, which often results in probation revocation and placement in residential facilities (NeMoyer et al., 2014). Residential juvenile justice placement has been

* The authors thank Philadelphia Family Court's Administrative Judge Margaret T. Murphy and Supervising Judge Walter J. Olszewski, Chief of Probation Services Faustino Castro-Jimenez, Deputy Chief of Probation Services Bennie Price, and current and former court administration and probation directors and staff, particularly Margaret Joyce, Miriam Prioleau, Amy Warner, and Cherae McWilliams for welcoming us into this partnership and collaborating to generate change to improve outcomes for youth under court supervision while maintaining community safety.

linked to negative outcomes for youth, including high recidivism and rearrest rates, decreased reenrollment in and graduation from school, reduced employment rates once released, and high rates of trauma and mental health concerns (Mendel, 2011). However, community-based juvenile justice programming that addresses youths' criminogenic needs, provides treatment for mental health and substance use issues, and recognizes frequent desistance from illegal behavior can promote young people's long-term success (Chung, Schubert, & Mulvey, 2007; Lipsey & Wilson, 1998).

The structure of the compliance-focused approach to juvenile probation case management often does not incorporate the substantial body of research on youths' development and decision-making capacities (for a review, see Goldstein, NeMoyer, Gale-Bentz, Levick, & Feierman, 2016). As a group, adolescents demonstrate substantial difficulties understanding legal requirements and appreciating the consequences of fulfilling—or failing to fulfill—expectations of the legal and probation systems, such as requirements to comply with probation conditions (Goldstein, Condie, Kalbeitzer, Osman, & Geier, 2003; Grisso et al., 2003). Their decision-making processes and resulting behaviors reflect a combination of neurological (Cauffman & Steinberg, 2000) and psychosocial factors (Cauffman et al., 2010) that affect their immaturity of judgment; due to such incomplete brain development, adolescents are particularly motivated by the short-term positive outcomes of decisions rather than the risks of long-term negative consequences (see Scott & Steinberg, 2008). Without recognizing and accounting for these developmental considerations, many aspects of traditional juvenile probation systems fail to optimally promote their success.

PURPOSE OF THE COLLABORATION

Between 2011 and 2015, Philadelphia's juvenile justice leaders established shared priorities to decrease rates of detention and placement, promote alternatives to out-of-home placement, integrate graduated sanctions into court supervision, and use research to inform and evaluate programming. Related efforts contributed to decreased numbers of detained youth, establishment of juvenile specialty courts (e.g., dependency-delinquency crossover court, juvenile treatment court, graduated sanctions court), and increased collaboration across city agencies via the Juvenile Detention Alternatives Initiative (JDAI) Collaborative Board and committees and Juvenile Justice System Enhancement Strategy (JJSES) statewide initiatives. There was an important remaining challenge, however: promoting youths' successful completion of probation.

There was consensus among juvenile justice agencies and organizations in Philadelphia (e.g., Family Court, Juvenile Probation Department, Department of Human Services [DHS], District Attorney's [DA's] Office, Defender Association, Police Department) about the importance of facilitating youths' successful completion of probation and providing the supports needed to keep youth out of the justice system whenever possible. Consistent with this goal, Philadelphia's Juvenile Probation Department began working through JDAI to expand the *Graduated Response* element of its approach to probation case management and system-wide implementation. Initially, this approach emphasized the use of graduated sanctions, using multiple sanctions prior to revoking probation and placing youth in out-of-home, residential settings. But despite the cross-system commitment to modifying probation practices to improve youth outcomes, it was necessary to have extensive discussions about the challenges of (1) revising policies and procedures to reflect empirically based principles and practices, (2) implementing such a paradigm shift in the system-level approach to juvenile probation case management, and (3) measuring the outcomes of these policy and practice changes. To address these gaps between research and practice, an academic–practice partnership was created between Dr. Naomi Goldstein's Juvenile Justice Research and Reform (JJR&R) Lab at Drexel University (referred to as "we" throughout) and key stakeholders in Philadelphia's juvenile justice community—primarily, Philadelphia's Juvenile Probation Department leadership and staff.

The purpose of this collaboration was to transform existing juvenile justice policy and practice into a structured system that emphasized and encouraged youths' successful completion of probation and long-term positive outcomes while enhancing public safety. To accomplish these goals, the partnership aimed to restructure organizational expectations of youth and revise policy and practice to align with research on adolescent development, best practices in youth behavior change, and principles of procedural justice. All of these fall under the umbrella of what we refer to as "Graduated Response."

Though we focus our discussion of Graduated Response as a specific case management approach for juvenile probation, the larger goal of the revised probation strategies was to establish a structured system that simultaneously set realistic expectations for and of youth, focused on improving youths' behavior rather than simply complying with court-ordered conditions, and emphasized individualized case planning with establishment of meaningful goals for supervised youth, with consistency in system execution across youth and juvenile probation officers (JPOs). As a case management approach, Graduated Response is empirically based and focuses on effectively changing the behavior of supervised youth through system-level policy and practice changes. Grounded in principles of operant conditioning, this developmentally informed approach uses incentives to promote positive behaviors and delivers targeted interventions to constructively address misbehavior at varying levels of seriousness. Importantly, Graduated Response systems shift the focus from reliance on sanctions for misbehavior to creation of opportunities for JPOs to conduct functional analyses of youths' misbehaviors in order to identify and deliver appropriate responses. Graduated Response is a product of translational research collaborations between academic researchers with expertise in adolescent development and behavior change and juvenile justice system practitioners with expertise in system operations and service delivery.

THE BEGINNINGS OF THE COLLABORATION

In 2011, the City of Philadelphia began participating in the Annie E. Casey Foundation-sponsored JDAI. Bringing together key stakeholders from multiple agencies and perspectives, Philadelphia's JDAI Collaborative Board (co-chaired by the Administrative Judge of Family Court and the Commissioner of the Department of Human Services and included representative leadership from the Juvenile Probation Department, Offices of the DA and Defender Association, and multiple other juvenile justice stakeholder groups in Philadelphia) authorized a qualitative and quantitative assessment of juvenile detention utilization at the time. As is common across the United States (Sickmund, Sladky, Kang, & Puzzanchera, 2011), many youth in detention and placement were there as a result of probation violations (e.g., missed school, failed drug screens, missed appointments) rather than new arrests (Mendel, 2009). Based on a review of data and the comprehensive system assessment, Philadelphia's JDAI Collaborative Board identified reforming juvenile probation practices to reduce violations of probation in order to reduce use of detention and placement as a priority.

To address this issue and proactively develop methods of reducing use of detention and placement, Philadelphia's Juvenile Probation Department created an interdisciplinary Task Force focused on reducing violations of probation and exploring more effective probation supervision structures, including Graduated Response. The Graduated Response Task Force was directed by Juvenile Probation leadership and included representatives from various juvenile justice agencies in the City, but it lacked a research-based perspective. Through existing partnerships with juvenile justice leaders in the City, Dr. Goldstein and the Chief of Juvenile Probation connected, and Dr. Goldstein received a fellowship from the Stoneleigh Foundation to join the Task Force and collaborate with Juvenile Probation Department and Family Court to develop and implement an empirically guided, developmentally informed Graduated Response system.

Financially, this project was initially supported through the Annie E. Casey Foundation's support of Philadelphia's JDAI and through the substantial in-kind resources of City of Philadelphia agencies in the form of staff time dedicated to Graduated Response development activities. The Stoneleigh Foundation supplemented these resources by supporting Dr. Goldstein's time to dedicate to this collaborative work. As Graduated Response development and implementation efforts continued, costs for incentives were built in, as a line item, to the Juvenile Probation Department's needs-based budget with the state.

SETTING UP THE COLLABORATION

After the Stoneleigh Fellowship was awarded to Dr. Goldstein, a Memorandum of Understanding (MOU) was established between the First Judicial District of Pennsylvania, Family Court, Philadelphia's Juvenile Probation Department, and

Drexel University, representing Dr. Goldstein and her JJR&R Lab. The MOU established the shared commitment to improving Philadelphia's juvenile probation system to make it more responsive to adolescent development and to foster youths' success on probation. The MOU also established expectations and agreements to prevent disclosure of confidential information owned and controlled by the Juvenile Probation Department. The JDAI Collaborative Board launched the Graduated Response Task Force, comprised of representatives from various City agencies and juvenile justice stakeholders. However, an important challenge soon became apparent: although all stakeholders' perspectives were needed to identify issues, the Juvenile Probation Department had primary control over many of the solutions. Therefore, a Graduated Response Committee of Juvenile Probation Department administration and staff began meeting on a monthly basis to explore possible Graduated Response approaches to juvenile probation supervision. Two members of our JJR&R Lab team joined this committee, and later, we co-staffed a small Working Group with senior Juvenile Probation staff to accelerate progress of the Graduated Response development process. Juvenile Probation administration, the Graduated Response Committee, and the Graduated Response Task Force reviewed documents created by the Working Group.

We worked with the Juvenile Probation Department over the course of several years of intensive development to create strategies, materials, and system structures that were data-driven, research-based, and reform-oriented. After the development of this system, we worked with the Juvenile Probation Department to jointly train staff, incorporate feedback, inform supervision, and provide consultation throughout the implementation process. This hands-on collaborative endeavor led the Juvenile Probation Department to incorporate research-informed principles into its policies and practices and to serve as a primary contributor to the statewide juvenile probation reform efforts. Together, we worked to establish policies and protocols to ensure the sustainability of the newly adopted Graduated Response approach to probation case management.

WHO IS INVOLVED

Many leaders, administrators, and staff were involved in the successful research–practice partnership between our team and the Juvenile Probation Department. At the local level, the City of Philadelphia's JDAI Collaborative Board served as the first organizing structure for situating the work within a broader network of system reform efforts. The Administrative Judge of Family Court, who served as co-chair of the JDAI Collaborative Board, supported the local probation reform initiatives and lent support to the Graduated Response project in particular. With the Administrative Judge's support, the incorporation of research components became central to the policy and practice changes in the prevention and management of probation violations and in using the Graduated Response approach to probation supervision.

At the state level, the Juvenile Court Judges' Commission (JCJC) and the Council of Chief Juvenile Probation Officers (Chiefs' Council) led the Graduated Response reform efforts across Pennsylvania and invited our team to sit on state-wide committees designed to facilitate the development and implementation of Graduated Response statewide and address associated system-level challenges (e.g., the need to restructure data management systems to align with Graduated Response practices). Additionally, in 2010, the Commonwealth of Pennsylvania adopted the JJSES to guide all juvenile probation practice across the state (PA Council of Chief Juvenile Probation Officers, 2019). JJSES emphasized that juvenile justice system practice should be informed by the best empirical research available in the field. Thus, the translational research approach used by the academic–practitioner partnership to develop Philadelphia's Graduated Response system aligned with state priorities. Graduated Response offered sustainable change, rather than a short-lived initiative championed by a single administrator, as it was adopted across multiple city- and statewide agencies and structures.

Stakeholders and administrators throughout the state had a meaningful role in supporting the changes implemented in county-level juvenile proba-tion departments; nevertheless, for the purposes of this chapter, we will focus on the reform efforts specific to Philadelphia's juvenile probation system. The Working Group, charged with system development and implementation, was made up of juvenile probation administrators, a JPO supervisor, the in-house JDAI coordinator, and members of our JJR&R Lab team. The Working Group was supported by and consistently received feedback and guidance from leaders of Philadelphia's Juvenile Probation Department. Additionally, the Working Group regularly presented progress to and received support and feedback from the JDAI Collaborative Board, including leadership from Family Court, as well as from leadership of other juvenile justice stakeholder agencies and organiza-tions, including DHS and the juvenile units of the Offices of the DA and Defender Association.

SERVICES DELIVERED

Because Graduated Response signified a major change to organizational policy and practice, it was important for the practitioners and academic researchers to work together on content. The messaging was then disseminated through written procedures, formulated documentation, and targeted in-person trainings. We had the necessary skills to facilitate focus groups with youth and JPOs to understand their perspectives on current case management practices and reform efforts; create documents that established clear, developmentally appropriate expectations and practices; lead training sessions focused on youth behavior and willingness to en-gage in a new probation approach; and provide consultation around early super-vision of JPOs as they began implementing the Graduated Response approach.

Consistent with best practice in the development and implementation of new system-wide services (Israel et al., 2018), evaluation at each stage was required.

Given our extensive experience evaluating novel justice-related programs, we were able to provide reports at each stage of the development process to the Working Group and Juvenile Probation Department administrators to guide decision-making. For example, we were able to create and administer assessments intended to evaluate JPOs' readiness to change and their understanding of the underlying principles of reform. Prior to and following each face-to-face Graduated Response training, we administered surveys to all participating JPOs to assess readiness for change; understanding and appreciation of Graduated Response principles, policies, and practices; potential challenges to system-wide implementation; and effectiveness of the training sessions. With the Graduated Response Working Group, we reviewed survey results and identified implications for further system refinement or training to promote a smooth transition to the new developmentally responsive probation strategy.

As part of the Working Group, we provided guidance on evaluating case management practices and measuring overall effectiveness of implementation across the department. Early in the implementation process, for instance, our collaborators at Juvenile Probation were concerned about JPOs implementing their newly learned case management practices reliably across the department. Using our research-based priority of maximizing fidelity to documented protocols, we assisted the Working Group with creating a supervision model to help JPOs consistently apply Graduated Response across youth on their caseloads. As part of the model, the Deputy Director of Juvenile Probation provided sample case plans and requested that the newly trained JPOs brainstorm short- and long-term goals and the action steps a youth might take to complete those goals. We supported the Deputy Director by offering reminders about the empirical basis for identifying goals and action steps to foster youths' positive behavior changes. JPOs were encouraged to ask questions specific to youth on their caseloads. Once JPOs met with youth, group supervision meetings were used to discuss the goals and action steps identified during meetings with youth and to address challenges that had arisen. For example, JPOs presented cases in which youth did not meet their identified short-term goals; the Deputy Director then led a discussion with JPOs and our team about potential reasons youth may not have met their goals (e.g., important action steps that were not specified, youths' competing interests, logistical obstacles to completion) and conducted role plays with the JPOs to help them address these concerns during their upcoming meetings with youth. Additionally, JPOs asked questions about how to present the progress of youth participating in the Graduated Response system on their caseloads to judges during regular court hearings.

It is important to recognize that although we came to the partnership with expertise in adolescent development and youth behavior change, as well as in research methods and fidelity monitoring, our goal was never to decide which particular outcomes were most important. The key system stakeholders involved in the collaboration needed to identify and prioritize objectives and evaluation questions—and *then* we provided consultation on effective approaches and methodology that would help achieve their aims and provide specific useful information. To that end, Juvenile Probation leadership identified two outcome areas of interest. First, they were interested in examining whether actual practices carried out by JPOs aligned with the expected practices of their newly established Graduated Response system. For example, given the research on effective behavior change (e.g., Kazdin, 1975; Power, Karustis, & Habbouche, 2001; Wodahl, Garland, Culhane, & McCarty, 2011), incentives and rewards should be given more frequently than interventions and consequences; probation staff members were interested in seeing if JPOs were doing this as intended. Second, Juvenile Probation leadership wanted to gauge the overall success of the new probation strategy compared to the previous model by examining the number of youth successfully completing probation, the amount of time spent on supervision, and the numbers of probation violations and youth detained or placed. A challenge arose, however, when we attempted to examine these questions because the data system used for case management was not designed with program evaluation and quality assurance considerations in mind. We offered consultation to both Philadelphia's Juvenile Probation Department, as well as to the Pennsylvania Graduated Response Data Committee, regarding how to capture data that would simultaneously support case management and program evaluation needs.

WHO IS SERVED

The collaboration between Philadelphia's Department of Juvenile Probation and the JJR&R Lab used a multilevel approach to change. The partnership aimed to change the policies, procedures, practices, and culture (i.e., attitudes and beliefs) of the overall Juvenile Probation Department (Level 1), as well as the practices, attitudes, and beliefs of individual JPOs (Level 2). By creating change at both Levels 1 and 2, we expected better outcomes for the individual youth on community supervision in Philadelphia (Level 3).

Level 1

Juvenile probation is typically structured as a compliance-based model in which youth are monitored for their adherence to court-mandated conditions (NeMoyer et al., 2014). If youth fail to fully comply with all court-ordered conditions (e.g., school attendance, curfew, clean drug screens, community service), JPOs or judges often respond by imposing sanctions. Although sanctions, particularly overly punitive sanctions, do not serve as an effective method of modifying adolescent behavior (Altschuler, 2005; Gershoff, 2002; Goldstein et al., 2016), most JPOs—in Philadelphia and elsewhere—relied heavily on the use of sanctions in their supervision of youth. Graduated Response, in contrast, focuses on using incentives to promote positive behavior and on identifying and addressing the underlying causes of negative behavior in order to promote youths' behavior change. Therefore, introducing developmentally and empirically informed strategies that encourage positive behavior; emphasize progress toward change over immediate, full compliance; and use a functional analysis approach to modify misbehavior required a shift in departmental policies, procedures, practices, and culture.

Level 2

The Juvenile Probation Department's system-level changes directly impacted the JPOs who interact with youth on a daily basis. Prior to Graduated Response, JPOs spent much of their time monitoring youths' compliance with probation conditions and seeking to modify misbehavior through formal or informal sanctions and restrictions. Of course, even before Philadelphia Juvenile Probation established the Graduated Response system, many JPOs extended their roles far beyond those of monitors or court officers to include case management and life coaching; nevertheless, the new system-wide approach formally structured JPOs' supervision of youth to expand the focus into broader areas of youths' lives. This was done both to identify and foster positive life goals and to understand and meaningfully address the underlying reasons for misbehavior. Additionally, Graduated Response procedures also encouraged JPOs to consider how best to elicit input from youth about their needs, promote goal-oriented positive behaviors, offer emotional and logistical support when needed, and recognize youths' attempts to practice new behavioral strategies. Beyond changing specific behaviors, JPOs reported that using the Graduated Response approach improved their relationships with many youth on their caseloads. For example, one JPO reported that when he began using Graduated Response procedures, the youth he supervised responded positively to his use of affirming feedback and his emphasis on helping them problem-solve different challenges in their lives. Not only did the youth feel supported by this probation officer, but the JPO noted that it was the first time he felt that he and his supervisees had overwhelmingly positive relationships.

Level 3

Although the collaboration focused on changing departmental policies and procedures and JPO practices, the goal of transitioning to a Graduated Response system was to improve youth outcomes while keeping communities safe. We hoped this would promote faster successful discharge from probation in the short-term and help youth acquire the skills and opportunities to promote their well-being, prevent recidivism, and stay out of the justice system in the long term. As recognized by the National Council of Juvenile and Family Court Judges (2017), the principles of Graduated Response practices, based in developmental research, can effect meaningful change in young people's lives on a daily basis as JPOs work with youth to set achievable short- and long-term goals, identify necessary action steps to complete such goals, and collaborate to problem-solve when goals are not accomplished. As the focus of supervision has shifted from monitoring youths' compliance with court conditions to analyzing the function of youths' behavior, youth are encouraged to work with their JPOs to brainstorm problem-solving strategies to achieve their goals. Youth mistakes (at least those not presenting a risk to community safety) thus can generate opportunities for growth rather than resulting in restrictive consequences such as in-home detention or probation revocation and placement. Such restrictions remove youth from their daily activities and prevent exposure to experiences in which learning occurs. The Graduated Response system aims to promote positive behavior change, improve decision-making skills, and facilitate the overall well-being of youth on probation—all while enhancing community safety by improving youth behavior, preventing recidivism, and providing youth with opportunities for long-term success.

HOW THE COLLABORATION FUNCTIONS

The collaboration between Philadelphia Juvenile Probation and the JJR&R Lab at Drexel University followed a model of community-based participatory action research (CBPAR), in which the experiences and expertise of all players are honored in order to create systemic changes (Stringer, 1996, 1999). Our designated role in this partnership was to share our expertise in juvenile justice program development, implementation, and evaluation so that juvenile justice stakeholders could create the content and programming that best met their goals given their extensive knowledge about the strengths, challenges, and needs of their system, staff, and youth. Therefore, the collaboration took different shapes across the various project stages.

As the Graduated Response development and implementation process was iterative, so, too, was the functioning of the collaboration. In the collaboration's early stages, much of the focus was on (1) identifying empirically based developmental, behavior change principles to guide general supervision strategies (e.g., use of incentives to promote positive behaviors) and (2) developing documents (e.g., tracking system for tangible incentives), policies and procedures (e.g., case management processes), and training materials for early implementation of the new system. Development was done collaboratively, with materials often created jointly by representatives of the Philadelphia Juvenile Probation Department and our team involved in the Graduated Response Working Group. These materials were then reviewed by the larger committee and administration; suggestions were provided, and the Working Group incorporated feedback into subsequent drafts. Given the significant work required to create all materials and strategize ways to shift organizational policy, the Working Group met in person twice weekly throughout the 3-year development stage, and ongoing work was conducted via email between meetings. The Working Group also met regularly with the larger Graduated Response Task Force to update the group regarding progress and plans and to seek feedback. Additionally, because Philadelphia's Graduated Response development and implementation efforts were conducted in conjunction with the broader set of reform strategies supported by JDAI, the Working Group held quarterly meetings with JDAI's Collaborative Board.

The Working Group re-examined aspects of Graduated Response development throughout the implementation stage as unanticipated challenges arose, such as the cumbersome nature of monitoring individual court conditions, as well as implementing a goal-based case plan (discussed in detail in a later section). In the final 2 years of the collaboration, the Working Group's focus largely shifted to the training and supervision of JPOs and supervisors. In this phase, we provided training on the empirically based foundational principles and core concepts of Graduated Response, and probation staff in the Working Group provided training on the "how to" of Philadelphia's Graduated Response system— for example, how to develop case plans with youth, how to use incentives and determine interventions in practice, and how to complete the new Graduated Response documents. The combination of our expertise in empirically based behavior change and adolescent development, and juvenile probation staff's applied expertise, provided a strong foundation for JPOs to begin utilizing the Graduated Response system.

Consistent with the CBPAR model (Becker, Israel, Gustat, Reyes, & Allen, 2013), the expectations of this partnership were to collaboratively create, implement, and promote the sustainability of structural change. Once the Graduated Response system was implemented successfully throughout the department, it was intended to be autonomously sustained by the Juvenile Probation Department. Several measures were taken to ensure the new approach's sustainability. First, all juvenile probation policies and documentation related to case management and monitoring were changed to reflect the Graduated Response model. Second, in addition to training all JPOs and supervisors in the theory and practice of Graduated Response, supervisors received supplemental training to establish their abilities to supervise JPOs in the new approach to case management. This supervisor training enhanced comfort with both the overall Graduated Response model and specific procedures for those responsible for overseeing JPOs' daily practices. The Working Group, with input from stakeholders in juvenile probation, recognized that Graduated Response practices could not exist solely in a juvenile probation silo. Accordingly, there were efforts to approach and train family court judges, staff at the DA's office, and public defenders to understand the language and requests of JPOs reporting on a youth's progress during court hearings and align their practices with the Graduated Response model. Such training sessions were led by members of the Working Group, including our Drexel research team and the Juvenile Probation Department's deputy directors. Finally, financial sustainability was considered; the Juvenile Probation Department moved from utilizing external grant funding to building financial support into its yearly needs-based budget with the state. Originally, the Juvenile Probation Department used external grant funding to support training and implementation costs of the Graduated Response model. However, recognizing the need to ensure financial sustainability of the initiative, the Juvenile Probation Department worked with the First Judicial District of Pennsylvania (juvenile court) to include Graduated

Response operating costs in it annual "Needs-Based Plan and Budget Estimate," the mechanism by which the State of Pennsylvania Department of Human Services provides financial support for local dependent and delinquent youth services.

SUCCESSFUL EXPECTATIONS AND AGREEMENTS

Much of the success of this collaboration can be attributed to the roles that were delineated early on by both sides of the partnership. We recognized that as academic researchers, we were not system partners; we acknowledged our comparative lack of applied experience in juvenile probation operations from the outset and continued to learn the distinct duties and expectations of those in juvenile probation throughout the collaboration. Without operational expertise or decision-making authority, we focused on our designated role: to identify core principles from adolescent development and behavior change research that would impact youths' capacities to successfully complete probation. We then provided the Juvenile Probation Workgroup with guidance on how to translate these core principles into policy and practice. Juvenile Probation staff members' roles were to merge our guidance with their extensive knowledge of the youth and system partners to determine how the core principles would translate into practice, always considering feasibility and balancing youth needs with community safety concerns.

Within this careful delineation of roles, the Juvenile Probation Department was very receptive. They opened their doors and files to our team and invited us to seek information about existing practices and raise questions to stimulate change. We were also encouraged to propose empirically based, developmentally informed probation practices and work with Juvenile Probation staff and administrators to translate those findings into policy, procedures, practice, and documentation.

In the spirit of CBPAR, we appreciated that the expertise of probation administration and staff is critical to developing and implementing a successful new strategy. Thus, we focused on those areas in which we could provide expertise, such as teaching methods to identify underlying reasons for misbehavior and creating outcome measurement tools. Recognizing and valuing the roles and unique contributions of each side of the partnership not only helped facilitate implementation of Graduated Response in Philadelphia; it also promoted the development of a trusting, long-term relationship between collaborators that allowed for fluid and nonjudgmental communication throughout all stages of the project and laid a foundation for future collaborations.

Despite the overall success of this collaboration in accomplishing the major system reform goal of implementing Graduated Response across all JPOs and youth in the department, we experienced challenges and learned several important lessons along the way, which we will take with us into future partnerships in Philadelphia and elsewhere. First, as translational researchers, we initially underestimated the difficulty in translating relevant research into practice at an operational level. For example, with the Working Group, we initially attempted to translate the power of affirmative feedback for positive behavior into the awarding of incentives for adherence to each court condition, as well as developing a case plan to identify short- and long-term goals and incentives to promote behavior change. But after piloting, it quickly became apparent that this was overwhelming for JPOs and youth, and it inadvertently emphasized monitoring compliance over proactive case planning and problem-solving. As a result, the Working Group, in collaboration with administration, decided to scale back the condition-specific monitoring and more strongly emphasize the use of the case plan to establish goals and constructively address challenges. Not only was this approach less cumbersome, but it also underscored JPOs' efforts to create opportunities for positive behavior change that would align with youths' individual goals. Second, we planned to provide continuous quality improvement feedback while implementing Graduated Response by using juvenile probation case management data. Unfortunately, once we had access to the database, we quickly discovered that the statewide data system did not yield the information needed to track real-time transformation—and database changes were outside local control. Thus, along with members of the Graduated Response Working Group, we joined the statewide Graduated Response Data Committee to develop long-term solutions to track implementation of system change and associated outcomes for county departments and the youth they serve and, in the meantime, relied on hard copy, Graduated Response documentation completed by Philadelphia JPOs in the course of their case management. This approach allowed for real-time feedback on implementation to the Juvenile Probation Department's Deputy Director overseeing Graduated Response supervision, and statewide work continues to revise the data system to provide more detailed data for outcome evaluation.

SIGNIFICANT CHANGES SINCE INCEPTION

There have been significant changes with respect to scope and emphasis since the inception of Graduated Response development in Philadelphia Juvenile Probation. Regarding scope, the Working Group conducted an initial field test and subsequent pilot testing with a limited number of JPOs, supervisors, and assistant supervisors prior to department-wide implementation. The initial field test was comprised of two JPOs who received training on the foundational principles, policies, and procedures of Graduated Response; each JPO implemented the approach with two to four youth and provided feedback on system successes and challenges to the Graduated Response Working Group. Using this feedback, the Working Group modified the existing policies and procedures to inform the pilot phase of Graduated Response implementation. During the pilot phase—which consisted of two rounds of pilot testing—a larger number of JPOs (10–15 per round), as well as all supervisors and assistant supervisors, received the updated training on the foundational principles, policies, and procedures; implemented the approach with 2–4 youth per JPO caseload; and participated in ongoing supervision by the Deputy Director of Juvenile Probation. Importantly, throughout this phase, JPOs completed Graduated Response documentation tracking forms, which were collected and reviewed by the Deputy Director to ensure program fidelity. At the conclusion of the pilot phase, the Graduated Response Working Group made additional revisions to the materials, policies, and procedures based on JPOs' feedback, information gleaned from the tracking forms, and analysis of preliminary outcome data. With revisions completed, training sessions for JPOs and supervisors continued. Following training, and supported by ongoing supervision, JPOs were expected to implement Graduated Response with *all* youth as they were added to their caseloads. As of Fall 2019, Graduated Response had been fully implemented throughout Philadelphia's Juvenile Probation Department, with all JPOs utilizing empirically based, developmentally informed practices that aim to promote positive behavior change with all youth placed on probation.

In addition to growth in the implementation of Graduated Response, significant changes regarding the emphasis of the system also occurred throughout the implementation phase. Initially, the Graduated Response approach focused on promoting youths' adherence to the conditions of probation. However, based on staff feedback and in line with changes occurring at the state level and with national efforts (e.g., NCJFCJ Resolution, 2017), the emphasis of Graduated Response in Philadelphia shifted to promoting youths' completion of short- and long-term goals identified in the case plan. A case plan document was created to record youths' short- and long-term goals, the action steps youth should complete in order to successfully reach their goals, and the incentives JPOs should provide for goal completion. Additionally, the Case Plan acted as a tracking document for youths' progress and for the incentives awarded in recognition of this progress. Unlike the previous—and typical—compliance-monitoring strategy, JPOs do not sanction youth who do not complete their goals; rather, JPOs work with youth to problem-solve, re-evaluate action steps, and modify goals as needed to promote youths' success and provide opportunities for growth.

Finally, given the immense changes to the structure of juvenile probation in Philadelphia, the Working Group has been viewed across the state as an example of a model for successful reform. For instance, a second Stoneleigh Fellowship was awarded to the JJR&R Lab to partner with JCJC and the Chiefs' Council to create a peer mentorship model involving teams of academic researchers and juvenile probation staff experienced with Graduated Response to assist Pennsylvania counties with developing and implementing their own systems. The Philadelphia Working Group members will serve as key contributors to these efforts, and the model will incorporate many aspects of the informal mentorship that Philadelphia Juvenile Probation staff members have already provided to other jurisdictions. Additionally, the materials and training sessions created in Philadelphia have been represented in statewide forums on Graduated Response and in developmentally informed case management strategies. Furthermore, Philadelphia's work has been reflected in national publications (e.g., Goldstein et al., 2019).

Over the course of 5 years, Graduated Response efforts spearheaded by the collaboration between the Philadelphia Juvenile Probation Department and JJR&R Lab at Drexel University have grown exponentially. All JPOs use Graduated

Response with all young people joining their caseloads. Given Philadelphia's role in contributing to statewide policy and offering mentorship to other jurisdictions, the Graduated Response efforts have had far-reaching effects.

MEASURING THE EFFECTIVENESS OF THE COLLABORATION

To shift from existing practices to Graduated Response, we aimed to achieve expectations at each stage of the process. These expectations, determined jointly by the Working Group, were developed to measure outcomes or provide deliverables. These could then be shared with others at local and state levels interested in Graduated Response. At the end of the development stage, our collaboration had established a set of policies and procedures for JPOs, supervisors, and administrators to follow in order to implement the Graduated Response model of juvenile probation. Additionally, materials and documents were created for practitioners to utilize on a daily basis (e.g., case plans, incentives tracking documents). For the implementation stage, Juvenile Probation leadership set the expectation that Graduated Response case management would serve as the supervision strategy across the department. Accordingly, with the Juvenile Probation members of the Working Group, we trained all 87 JPOs, about 15 at a time, and 18 supervisors and assistant supervisors (using the same 2-day principles and practices training in order to promote fidelity). These trained JPOs are currently using Graduated Response with all 1,300 youth currently on juvenile probation in Philadelphia. Finally, as part of our efforts to evaluate the success of system implementation, we assessed changes in JPOs' (1) willingness to change and (2) knowledge and attitudes about youth behavior, development, and behavior change using pre- and post-training surveys. Having a streamlined way to quantitatively evaluate the success of Graduated Response by examining overall numbers of youth who successfully complete probation involves ongoing collaboration with statewide committees. Specifically, we are working to change the online case management data system to provide easily accessible outcome data to all jurisdictions that have implemented Graduated Response.

LESSONS LEARNED AND IMPLICATIONS

Throughout this collaboration, we learned important lessons about how to create academic–practitioner collaborations to generate meaningful, sustainable juvenile justice reform. Most importantly, our successful partnership with Philadelphia's Juvenile Probation Department reinforced the value of strong and trusting relationships between collaborators. Initially, before we had the opportunity to get to know one another as individuals and create strong interpersonal relationships, it was critical to establish clear expectations about the roles and responsibilities of each individual and entity. Over time, we were able to develop trust; as questions and concerns arose, we always brought them directly to the Juvenile Probation Department, and they brought them directly to us. When development processes became difficult or tense—as they inevitably do with large-scale change—we never walked away from the collaboration, and they welcomed us to their table twice each week. We all established that this partnership represented a long-term commitment, and, as a Working Group, we consistently reminded ourselves that we were working toward the shared goal of producing better outcomes for youth on probation.

Additionally, through this Graduated Response partnership, we learned several lessons to guide our future academic–practitioner collaborations designed to produce large-scale juvenile justice change. First, we learned the importance of flexibility in designing and implementing major system reform, drawing on rapid-cycle improvement theory and methodology (Lewis, 2015): based on information produced during the field test and each of the pilot trials, the Working Group revisited system priorities and revised policies and procedures to create a more feasible and effective system. Second, we learned the value of understanding from the beginning how local system-change efforts align with changes taking place at the state and national levels; the Graduated Response work in Philadelphia benefited from alignment with state Graduated Response efforts and national reforms (e.g., NCJFCJ, 2017). Third, this partnership and work benefited from the early creation of a sustainability plan. From the inception of this academic–practitioner collaboration, the intensity of the joint work was designed to decrease over time and, following training of the final set of JPOs, transition exclusively to the Juvenile Probation Department. Additionally, recognizing that personnel changes occur over time, the Working Group, with guidance from Juvenile Probation administration and other stakeholders, institutionalized these reforms by creating training documents for use with new JPOs, memorializing Graduated Response philosophy and practice in departmental policies and procedures, and incorporating the Graduated Response approach into the practice of multiple justice agencies.

The successful implementation of this large-scale, empirically based juvenile justice system reform directly impacts the experiences of the more than 1,000 youth under probation supervision in Philadelphia and establishes a model for other jurisdictions seeking change. Furthermore, this successful academic–practitioner partnership and lessons learned creates a strong foundation from which to generate future system change.

REFERENCES

Altschuler, D. M. (2005). Policy and program perspectives on the transition to adulthood for adolescents in the juvenile justice system. On your own without a net: The transition to adulthood for vulnerable populations, 92–113.

Becker, A., Israel, B., Gustat, J., Reyes, A., & Allen, A. (2013). Strategies and techniques for effective group process in CBPR partnerships. In B. Israel, E. Eng, A. Schulz, &

E. Parker (Eds.), *Methods for community-based participatory research for health* (pp. 69–96). San Francisco: Wiley.

Cauffman, E., Shulman, E. P., Steinberg, L., Claus, E., Banich, M. T., Graham, S., & Woolard, J. (2010). Age differences in affective decision making as indexed by performance on the Iowa Gambling Task. *Developmental Psychology, 46*(1), 193–207.

Cauffman, E., & Steinberg, L. (2000). (Im)maturity of judgment in adolescence: Why adolescents may be less culpable than adults. *Behavioral Sciences & the Law, 18,* 741–760.

Chung, H. L., Schubert, C. A., & Mulvey, E. P. (2007). An empirical portrait of community reentry among serious juvenile offenders in two metropolitan cities. *Criminal Justice and Behavior, 34,* 1402–1426.

Gershoff, E. T. (2002). Corporal punishment by parents and associated child behaviors and experiences: A meta-analytic and theoretical review. *Psychological Bulletin, 128*(4), 539–579.

Goldstein, N. E., Condie, L. O., Kalbeitzer, R., Osman, D., & Geier, J. (2003). Juvenile offenders' *Miranda* rights comprehension and self-reported likelihood of offering false confessions. *Assessment, 10,* 359–369.

Goldstein, N. E., Gale-Bentz, E., McPhee, J., NeMoyer, A., Walker, S., Bishop, S., ... Schwartz, R. G. (2019). Applying the National Council of Juvenile and Family Court Judges' resolution to juvenile probation reform. *Translational Issues in Psychological Science, 5*(2), 170.

Goldstein, N. E., NeMoyer, A., Gale-Bentz, E., Levick, M., & Feierman, J. (2016). You're on the right track: Using graduated response systems to address immaturity of judgment and enhance youths' capacities to successfully complete probation. *Temple Law Review, 88,* 803–836.

Grisso, T., Steinberg, L., Woolard, J., Cauffman, E., Scott, E., Graham, S., ... Schwartz, R. (2003). Juveniles' competence to stand trial: A comparison of adolescents' and adults' capacities as trial defendants. *Law and Human Behavior, 27,* 333–363.

Hockenberry, S. & Puzzanchera, C. (2018). *Juvenile Court Statistics 2015.* Pittsburgh, PA: National Center for Juvenile Justice. https://www.ojjdp.gov/ojstatbb/publications/StatBBAbstract.asp?BibID=273908

Israel, B. A., Shulz, A. J., Parker, E. A., Becker, A. B., Allen III, A. J., Guzman, R., & Lichtenstein, R. (2018). Critical issues in developing and following CBPR principles. In N. Wallerstein, B. Duran, J. Oetzel, & M. Minkler (Eds.), *Community-based participatory research for health* (3rd ed.). San Francisco: Wiley.

Kazdin, A. E. (1975). *Behavior modification in applied settings.* Long Grove, IL: Waveland Press.

Lewis, C. (2015). What is improvement science? Do we need it in education? *Educational Researcher, 44*(1), 54–61.

Lipsey, M. W., & Wilson, D. B. (1998). Effective intervention for serious juvenile offenders: A synthesis of research. In R. Loeber & D. P. Farrington (Eds.), *Serious and violent juvenile offenders: Risk factors and successful interventions* (pp. 313–345). Thousand Oaks, CA: Sage.

Mendel, R. A. (2009). *Two decades of JDAI: From demonstration project to national standard.* Baltimore, MD: Annie E. Casey Foundation, Juvenile Detention Alternatives Initiative.

Mendel, R. A. (2011). *No place for kids: The case for reducing juvenile incarceration.* http://www.aecf.org/~/media/Pubs/Topics/Juvenile%20Justice/Detention%20Reform/NoPlaceForKids/JJ_NoPlaceForKids_Full.pdf

National Council of Juvenile and Family Court Judges [NCJFCJ]. (2017). *NCJFCJ resolves to help modernize approach to juvenile probation with better understanding of adolescent brain development* [Press release]. http://www.ncjfcj.org/Juvenile-Probation-Resolution

NeMoyer, A., Goldstein, N. E., McKitten, R. L., Prelic, A., Ebbecke, J., Foster, E., & Burkard, C. (2014). Predictors of juveniles' noncompliance with probation requirements. *Law and Human Behavior, 38*(6), 580–591.

PA Council of Chief Juvenile Probation Officers (2019). JJSES: Juvenile Justice System Enhancement Strategy. https://pachiefprobationofficers.org/jjses.php

Power, T. J., Karustis, J. L., & Habboushe, D. F. (2001). *Homework success for children with ADHD: A family-school intervention program.* New York: Guilford.

Scott, E. S., & Steinberg, L. (2008). *Rethinking juvenile justice.* Cambridge, MA: Harvard University Press.

Sickmund, M., Sladky, T. J., Kang, W., & Puzzanchera, C. (2011). *Easy access to the Census of Juveniles in Residential Placement* [Data file]. Washington, DC: US Department of Justice, Office of Justice Programs, Office of Juvenile Justice and Delinquency Prevention. http://www.ojjdp.gov/ojstatbb/ezacjrp/

Stringer, E. T. (1996). *Action research: A handbook for practitioners.* Thousand Oaks, CA: Sage.

Stringer, E. T. (1999). *Action research: A handbook for practitioners* (2nd ed.). Thousand Oaks, CA: Sage.

Wodahl, E. J., Garland, B., Culhane, S. E., & McCarty, W. P. (2011). Utilizing behavioral interventions to improve supervision outcomes in community-based corrections. *Criminal Justice and Behavior, 38*(4), 386–405.

9

University–Public Behavioral Health Collaboration

The Florida Mental Health Institute

KATHLEEN MOORE, JOSHUA T. BARNETT, ANNETTE CHRISTY,
MARIE MCPHERSON, AND MELISSA CARLSON ■

The Louis de la Parte Florida Mental Health Institute (FMHI) has engaged policy-makers, advocates, researchers, practitioners, and consumers to improve services for individuals with mental health conditions and intellectual disabilities for more than 45 years. Its mission to improve the lives of people with mental, addictive, and developmental disorders is accomplished through research and evaluation, policy advice, training, and technical assistance that is provided within Florida but also throughout the world. FMHI works broadly to strengthen the systems that support individuals of all ages who are engaged by behavioral health, criminal justice, child welfare, or other social welfare services. Seated within the College of Behavioral and Community Sciences at the University of South Florida (USF), FMHI has evolved from its original vision as a modern community health facility in the 1970s to becoming a leader in research, policy, and practice for children and adults with behavioral health needs (College of Behavioral and Community Science, 2017). FMHI's evolution aligns with national policy changes, which includes identifying emerging needs. Three of FMHI's collaborations are described in this chapter. These projects include the collection and reporting of involuntary psychiatric examinations completed throughout Florida, a state Medicaid drug therapy management program, and research partnerships with multiple problem-solving specialty courts.

FMHI was developed following actions by President John F. Kennedy that signaled the beginning of the community mental health center movement and the phasing out of large state psychiatric hospitals in the early 1960s (Community Mental Health Centers Construction Act [CMHA], 1963). As national policy focused on the deinstitutionalization of people treated in large, costly psychiatric treatment facilities, the 1967 Florida Legislature allocated $16 million for the construction of a mental health facility to be located in Tampa, Florida. Located on approximately 43 acres of the USF campus, FMHI officially opened its doors in 1974. The purpose of FMHI was to blend elements of service, research, and training; it would serve as a connection between state hospitals and community health centers, providing university-based research for professionals and communities addressing mental illness. By 1976, FMHI's defined mission was to train mental health professionals; conduct research on the causes, care, and prevention of mental health problems; and provide treatment options to individuals in need. Through dedication to this mission, FMHI became Florida's principal facility for mental health resources. Since then, through advances in national and state behavioral health policy, along with actions that made FMHI part of the state university system, FMHI has continued to provide high-impact research and training. Since 1996, FMHI is renamed the Louis de la Parte Florida Mental Health Institute, in honor of the Florida legislator who played a key role in establishing FMHI.

Although physically located on university property, FMHI was originally considered the property of the state's mental health authority, which was housed in what was then known as the Florida Department of Health and Rehabilitative Services (HRS). The HRS division director of mental health in the early 1960s requested the creation of a 500-bed facility to ease crowding in state hospitals, which were all located in towns that were rural at the time (Arcadia, Chattahoochee, Macclenny, and Pembroke Pines.) A needs assessment, completed by the American Psychiatric Association in 1963, reported that Hillsborough County led the rest of Florida for involuntary commitments of persons to mental health facilities (Division of Mental Health of the Department of HRS, 1969;). These findings, in addition to the medical complex at the USF, ultimately resulted in the decision that Tampa would receive one of four such facilities (*Tampa Times*, 1965, p. 1). FMHI's location was selected for Tampa's larger population, which at the time was considered urban, with 397,000 residents in Hillsborough County. Tampa could provide greater opportunities to recruit physicians and serve more people compared to other metropolitan areas of Florida.

Mental health leaders throughout Florida were in agreement that an urban location on the populous west coast was needed; however, political controversy and competing needs nearly disrupted the new location on two occasions. Rural legislators from Hernando County, 44 miles north of Tampa, wanted to house the new mental health facility as it would generate jobs for their community. Advocates of the more urban location in Tampa included the Florida Mental Health Association's president-elect, Dr. Moke Wayne Williams, who protested that a decision to build elsewhere would "set our mental health program back to those snake-pit and human warehouse days—bricks without brains" (Cribb, 1966, p. 2). Soon after the first request to reconsider the location, legislator Maxine E. Baker of Miami-Dade County filed a bill to have the facility located in her district, where she proposed it would become a teaching facility at the University of Miami. A compromise was reached and plans for FMHI continued with a renewed commitment to build in Tampa.

The state's HRS director of mental health, Dr. Rogers, presented innovative construction plans as part of the "bold new approach" he had envisioned for the institute. The futuristic design created yet another threat to the development of FMHI in 1969 when met with competing costs for other university expansions. State Senator Louis de la Parte of Tampa successfully secured the funding in the 1970 legislature, incorporating the provision that the institute would provide outpatient care to those who could not afford it. Modifications to Dr. Rogers's vision were required because appropriated funds were less than the construction plans required. Dr. E. Arthur Larson, a psychiatrist and mental health reformer, was selected to oversee these modifications. Dr. Larson sought to prevent FMHI from becoming a state hospital that would house people with mental illness and went so far as to reconfigure the structure in ways that would prevent the facility from ever meeting state hospital building standards.

Once construction was complete, in 1974, FMHI began to provide inpatient and outpatient psychiatric treatment services, partial hospitalization, emergency mental health care, and clinical diagnostic services. New and innovative treatment methods were also tested on site with the goal of improving staff training and performance in mental health facilities throughout Florida. In addition, FMHI facilitated community education initiatives and partnered with the USF School of Medicine to train psychiatrists, psychologists, and other professionals in mental health–related topics. FMHI modeled its integrative approach after existing university-based research and training sites like those located at the University of California and the State University of New York. Once opened, FMHI expanded in 1976 to include children's services and an updated activities center.

The 1980s was a decade of milestones and accomplishments for FMHI. In 1982, its first director, Dr. Jack Zusman, was recruited and provided with authority equivalent to that of a dean at USF. In 1983, citizen groups concerned with mental health services prevailed on the legislature to transfer FMHI from the Florida Department of Health and Rehabilitative Services to USF. When FMHI was transferred to USF, Dr. Zusman as director then reported to USF president as if FMHI were a college in the university. The 1984 budget prepared by the Governor's office eliminated all funding for FMHI. This same year, the legislature enacted sweeping changes to the Florida Mental Health Act (also known as the "Baker Act"). It was only through advocacy and support from citizen groups and from USF that the legislature restored funding for FMHI.

Several new FMHI Centers were developing during this tumultuous time for mental health policy. In 1984, a federally funded Research and Training Center for Children's Mental Health was developed to address the need for improved services for children and adolescents with severe emotional disturbances and their families. The Center for Autism and Related Disabilities (CARD) was also established in 1984. In 1987, the Juvenile Justice Training Academy and the Residential Aging Project both commenced. Last, in 1988, the Center for HIV Education and Research was established to provide education and training to healthcare professionals serving HIV/AIDS patients.

In 1988, the Florida Legislature appointed a task force to "review the role of state-sponsored research in the area of mental health services and evaluate the mission of FMHI specifically as it related to research and service delivery." Former state senator Louis de la Parte agreed to chair this task force; this same year, Dr. Max Dertke was hired as the new dean of FMHI.

By the 1990s, the field of mental health had evolved to focus more on the delivery of care in the community than in hospitals. This shift instigated a change in research focus and an increased emphasis on the development of public policy for Florida and the nation. As part of the new policy focus, FMHI was asked by the Florida Legislature to help revise the state's involuntary civil commitment law, known as the Baker Act. This legislative request provided FMHI with opportunities to study the issue of insurance parity and its financial impacts to the state's budget, treat mental health and substance use conditions, help revise the children's mental health state code, and evaluate strategies to finance mental health treatment and supports. Also, at this time, FMHI began to offer its own courses as part of a new graduate certificate program at USF. By 1995, the significant change in focus and the expanding opportunities for impact in the field also brought with it a new director, Dr. David Shern. In 1996, FMHI was renamed the Louis de la Parte FMHI by the Florida Legislature to honor the contributions of the state senator and former Senate president who focused on juvenile justice, mental health, and education prior to his death in 2008.

Dr. Bob Friedman was appointed as Interim Dean of FMHI in 2006, followed by the permanent appointment of Dr. Junius Gonzalez as Dean in 2007. FMHI implemented its first intensive Summer Research Institute (SRI) through a National Science Foundation (NSF) grant under the leadership of the Associate Dean. The SRI was developed to encourage undergraduate seniors to pursue research in behavioral health by providing opportunities to conduct community-based research under faculty mentorship. In 2012, we applied for and were awarded 5 years of additional funding from the National Institute of Mental Health (NIMH) for essentially the same summer program (major changes included attending 10 weeks instead of 9, a greater focus on mental health issues, and the addition of a high school component) and completed the NIMH grant in 2017. In 2018, we applied for our third round of SRI funding through the National Institute of Drug Abuse (NIDA) and received funding for another 5 years with a focus on addiction and co-occurring disorders. The Criminal Justice Mental Health and Substance Abuse Technical Assistance Center was established in 2007 to provide assistance to communities who received Department of Children and Families (DCF) reinvestment grants to fund justice system diversions for adults and children with behavioral health disorders. This same year, the Center for Child Welfare was established to support and strengthen best practices in the state's child welfare system. Perhaps the largest changes for FMHI came in 2008, when it became part of the newly formed College of Behavioral and Community Sciences (CBCS) at USF. CBCS is grounded in the same founding principles as FMHI and remains focused on advancing knowledge though interdisciplinary training, research, and services to improve the capacity of individuals, families, and diverse communities for living productive, satisfying, healthy, and safe lives. FMHI changed from being defined as a collection of departments at USF to an affiliate model, where faculty and staff from other departments at USF and community partners can become "affiliates" of FMHI and benefit from the collaboration provided by a College partnership.

In 2011, Dr. Larry Schonfeld was appointed Interim Executive Director of FHMI. Dr. Mary Armstrong became FMHI's first female Executive Director in 2014. Dr. Armstrong led FMHI in providing the Governor with a comprehensive review of local, state, and federally funded behavioral health services and an analysis of how well these services were integrated with other community services. An annual FMHI Fall Community Colloquium was developed to gather experts and local community leaders to discuss contemporary issues including mental health, guns, and violence; the effects of incarceration on offenders, families, and communities; and the intersection between the mental health and criminal justice systems. The CBCS Dean appointed Dr. Kathleen Moore as FMHI's sixth Executive Director in 2018.

FMHI and its affiliates continue to focus on some of society's most critical issues through research, consultation, and collaboration. At this time, more than $12 million in grants and contracts support FMHI's interdisciplinary work in the areas of psychology, psychiatry, economics, criminology, gerontology, anthropology, social work, public health, nursing, and education. FMHI now houses Florida's largest professional development center for the training of child welfare workers, training more than 6,000 child welfare and juvenile justice staff members annually. Florida KIDS COUNT is housed within FMHI and is the state's repository of statistical data for indicators of child well-being. The Child and Family Studies Department is host to the International Conference on Positive Behavior Support, the largest conference devoted to the support of children and families, with nearly 1,300 annual attendees, and the Annual Research and Policy Conference on Child, Adolescent, and Young Adult Behavioral Health. FMHI's Baker Act Reporting Center (BARC), in the Department of Mental Health Law and Policy, receives and analyzes involuntary examination documents for both children and adults from all of the more than 100 Baker Act receiving facilities statewide.

FMHI continues its mission to strengthen mental health and substance use services on behalf of individuals and communities that are impacted by these challenges. It is through the research and evaluation studies of its affiliates, as well as the training, technical assistance, policy formation, and stakeholder engagement that the mission of FMHI is accomplished. Throughout its history and development, FMHI has thrived because of its collaborative work with community leaders, national research partnerships, and integrative initiatives supporting state agencies like the Departments of Children and Families (DCF), Corrections (DOC), Education (DOE), Elder Affairs (DOEA), Juvenile Justice (DJJ), and the Agency for Health Care Administration (AHCA).

BAKER ACT REPORTING CENTER

Purpose and Collaboration

All states and the District of Columbia allow for short-term, involuntary assessment and treatment of persons with mental illness (Hedman, Petrila, Fisher, Swanson, Dingman, & Burris, 2016). An interactive database of national short-term emergency commitment laws is available at the Policy Surveillance Program (2016; also see Substance Abuse and Mental Health Services Administration [SAMHSA], 2019, for additional information on historical trends and principles for law and practice of civil commitment). This Florida statute (F.S. 394, Part I) is known as the Baker Act, named after Maxine Baker, the legislator who was the primary author of the original act in 1971. The Baker Act includes requirements for both voluntary and involuntary examination and treatment. Baker Act examinations, or "short-term involuntary examinations," may be initiated by law enforcement officers, certain health professionals, and by ex-parte order of a judge upon evidence of (a) mental illness, (b) harm to self, harm to others, and/ or self-neglect, and (c) refusal of treatment and/or lack of competence to consent to treatment. The Baker Act allows for people who meet these criteria to be held involuntarily for up to 72 hours in one of the more than 100 Florida DCF-designated Baker Act receiving facilities, where all Baker Act involuntary examinations occur. It also allows for longer term civil commitment, termed "involuntary inpatient placement" and "involuntary outpatient services," which can be initiated by the administrator of a Baker Act receiving facility by submitting a petition to the Clerk of Court.

When and Why the Collaboration Began

The Baker Act Reporting Center (BARC) was established in 1997 as the result of changes to the statute that came about, in part, because of a newspaper series that focused on the problematic use of Baker Act examinations for older adults (Marbin & Nohlgren, 1995a–e). This change called for more accountability and process transparency by requiring Baker Act receiving facilities statewide to submit the forms used to initiate involuntary examinations to the Florida AHCA. The BARC was established to receive and process these forms for AHCA. The requirements for facilities to submit forms to the BARC are not included directly in the statute. Submission of forms to the BARC is described in the Florida Administrative Code (F.A.C. 65E-5; Florida Administrative Code, 2019). A statutory change took effect in July 2016 (SB12, 2016), such that the BARC now receives these documents on behalf of DCF instead of AHCA and also receives petitions and orders for longer term (inpatient and outpatient) civil commitment from clerks of court statewide. The documents received by the BARC are listed in Table 9.1.

Table 9.1 INVOLUNTARY EXAMINATION, INPATIENT PLACEMENT, AND OUTPATIENT
SERVICES DOCUMENTS RECEIVED AT THE BAKER ACT REPORTING CENTER

Florida Department of Children and Families (DCF) (1998) CF-MH 3118	Cover Sheet to Department of Children and Families Completed by Baker Act receiving facility staff and included with each 3052a, 3052b and 3001 form

Forms Used to Initiate Involuntary (Baker Act) Examinations (since 1997)

DCF (2016a) CF-MH 3052a	Report of Law Enforcement officer Initiating Involuntary Examination
DCF (2016b) CF-MH 3052b	Certificate of Professional Initiating Involuntary Examination
DCF (2016c) CF-MH 3001	Ex-Parte Order for Involuntary Examination

Documents Used in the Involuntary Inpatient Placement& Outpatient Services Process (since 2018)

DCF (2005a) CF-MH 3032	Petition for Involuntary Inpatient Placement
DCF (2005b) CF-MH 3008	Order for Involuntary Inpatient Placement
DCF (2005c) CF-MH 3130	Petition for Involuntary Outpatient Placement
DCF (2006) CF-MH 3145	Proposed Individualized Treatment Plan for Involuntary Outpatient Placement or Continued Involuntary Outpatient Placement
DCF (2005d) CF-MH 3155	Order for Involuntary Outpatient Placement or Continued Outpatient Placement

How the Collaboration Functions

BARC Current Operations. The BARC has statewide client-identified, encounter-level data for short-term involuntary examinations and, as of 2018, for longer term civil commitment to inpatient and outpatient services. There were 210,992 Baker Act examinations in Fiscal Year 2018–2019 (Christy, Rhode, & Jenkins, 2020). The volume of forms received to date for Fiscal Year 2018–2019, in combination with data from the Office of State Court Administrators (Florida Courts, 2019), suggests that the BARC may receive between 35,000 and 50,000 petitions and orders for longer term civil commitment from clerks of court for the year.

Challenges and Considerations. Handling and entering data from more than 200,000 documents annually is costly. Some forms for involuntary examination submitted by Baker Act receiving facilities are still sent via US mail. The BARC has developed a system over the past 3 years for Baker Act receiving facilities and clerks of court to securely transfer scanned documents to the BARC using Box.com (a secure document management and storage system that is compliant with Health Insurance Portability and Accountability Act [HIPAA]) or using a Secure File Transfer Protocol. All clerks of court and the majority of the Baker Act receiving facilities are now using these electronic means of transfer in lieu of mailing documents. The BARC benefits from being in a university environment by using USF IT technical assistance as well as space on USF SQL and SFTP servers, as well as USF's instance of Box.com to implement the transition of Baker Act receiving facilities to secure, electronic transfer of forms at no additional cost to the BARC.

The documents submitted to the BARC were not originally created for the purpose of data collection or research, but rather to serve as legal documentation for involuntary assessment and/or treatment. Having standardized forms is essential to ensure all legal requirements are addressed. These forms have also helped to standardize data collection and data entry. The templates for the documents received at the BARC are part of the DCF Baker Act rule (Florida Administrative Code, 65E-5, 2019) and the forms can only be changed through the administrative rule promulgation process. While this process limits the ability to make rapid changes to forms, it provides a standardized means for key stakeholders to provide input for rule language and form revision (see Florida Statutes 120, Florida Administrative Procedures Act, 2019, and Joint Administrative Procedures Committee, n.d.).

The goal is for variables to be added to the forms only if the majority of people completing them could reasonably have the information for that variable. For example, adding a variable indicating whether a youth has an Individualized Education Plan (IEP) has been suggested. However, it is not likely that law enforcement completing the CF-MH3052a form or staff at the Baker Act receiving facility completing the Cover Sheet (CF-MH3118) will have this information. The length of forms needs to be minimized so that necessary information can be provided without an undue time burden.

The BARC has created a proof-of-concept to DCF for the formatting and use of machine-readable forms. After an initial up-front cost to implement and then a smaller cost per year to run, the use of machine-readable forms holds promise for more timeliness of data processing and quality checking of data, as well as reduced labor costs.

Changes to electronic submission and the machine reading of forms are important to our university–public behavioral health partnership because they will allow us to (a) make better use of the public resources provided to us by the state and (b) improve the logistics and reduce the cost for certain types of research we have been wanting to pursue. For example, the system for machine-reading forms can provide a link in each row of data to the form from which the data from that involuntary examination were entered. This will make qualitative coding of the forms much easier, minimizing the labor needed create a separate PDF document for each involuntary examination as required by software such as atlas.ti. DCF would benefit by our enhanced ability to be able to provide lower cost and more timely access to images of the forms.

Rules and Regulations

The statutory requirement for submission of documents is essential to the success ·
of the BARC. Since receiving facilities and clerks of court are faced with many
operational responsibilities, they might be less likely to submit documents if their
submission were not mandatory. The specificity written into the rule (F.A.C. 65E-
5) provides instructions for carrying out the statute but also describes the intent
of the process: holding all parties accountable under formalized and standardized
expectations. The BARC is also required by contract to send biannual compliance
reports to mandated reporters (Baker Act receiving facilities and clerks of court),
which promotes transparency and allows BARC staff to spend time addressing
compliance issues.

Understanding the Data

It is important for those using information from the BARC forms to understand
what the data are and what they are not, which is continually highlighted in
discussions with key stakeholders and in reports. For example, the BARC involuntary examination data do not tell us if a person was admitted, only whether an
involuntary examination was initiated. Also, the BARC does not receive forms
for voluntary admissions, which means that BARC data cannot provide the total
number of people who presented at a Baker Act unit for acute care.

Contractual Details

The BARC had no dedicated state funding from 1997 until July 2016. The BARC
was funded with USF resources such as (a) university-funded salaries using state
dollars, (b) salary savings, (c) the department's portion of the indirect/Facilities
&Administration (F&A) from externally funded projects, (d) federal work study
student time, and (e) a Medicaid research contract between USF and the AHCA.
The BARC crafted research projects for this AHCA contract in a way that allowed
for a portion of BARC data processing to be funded. With university budget cuts
beginning in the mid-2000s due to the economic downturn, the funding that had
previously been available to support the BARC was instead used to support staff
positions that had previously been funded by state (university) dollars, salary savings, and indirect funds. The BARC's financial standing improved when new statutory language took effect in July 2016 that changed the agency for which the
BARC received forms from the mid-1990s from AHCA to the Florida DCF. The
BARC is currently funded via a 5-year contract with the state of Florida using
a combination of state and federal (block grant) funds. As USF does not allow
the co-mingling of state and federal funds, this necessitates two budgets: one for
state funds and one for federal funds. This USF requirement calls for additional

coordination with our accounting staff. The BARC has been able to enter data within 30 days of form receipt because of this improved funding. The 5-year length of the BARC's current contract allowed the hiring of staff who can now rely on stable positions. These new staff positions include a full-time manager who assists the BARC Director with the day-to-day operations, as well as a part-time programmer. The BARC has been able to produce a larger annual report since 2017.

The university setting and the limited availability of funds to maintain full-time dedicated data processing staff positions means that the BARC relies mostly on part-time data processing staff, many of whom are university students or recent graduates. This includes part-time hourly paid staff, as well as Federal Work Study (FWS) student time. The FWS time is offered by the University at no cost to the project, a benefit to the state from this university partnership. The BARC must plan for limited availability of student-staff time during finals, semester breaks, summer break, and the closure of USF over each winter holiday. This presents a challenge given the contractual requirement to stay within 30 days up to date with data entry. Conveying to stakeholders what the BARC costs to run and thrive is an ongoing effort.

How Effectiveness Is Measured

The existence of the BARC has allowed the use of data to inform policy, the provision of services, and the implementation of statute and rule. This includes (a) assisting DCF to meet its statutory reporting requirements (see Christy, Rhode & Jenkins, 2020) and (b) providing data to inform the activities of legislative sessions. The BARC assists DCF to produce a report of repeated Baker Act examinations of children that is statutorily required as of 2019 (SB1418, 2019; Florida Department of Children and Families, 2019). The Baker Act data were used to inform a short-term legislatively created DCF Task Force on Baker Act Examinations of Minors (Florida Department of Children and Families, 2017) and reports of legislative committees (Florida Senate, 2004, 2005). More than 200 ad hoc reports of Baker Act data have been produced over the past two decades, addressing requests from media and a variety of other community stakeholders.

The Marchman Act (Florida Statutes 397, 2019) specifies how people can be involuntarily ordered to evaluation and treatment for substance abuse. At the request of DCF, BARC staff have also described what would be required to create a Marchman Act data system modeled on the Baker Act system so this can be considered by the Florida legislature. The analysis of the longer term civil commitment data from petitions and orders will be an important addition to the BARC reporting. While the Baker Act receiving facility system differs from how many other states handle short-term involuntary examinations, the Baker Act data can still be used to address issues in a way that is generalizable beyond Florida (Catalano, Kessell, Christy, & Monahan, 2005; Kessell, Catalano, Christy, & Monahan, 2006).

Services Delivered

Each business day the BARC staff, on average, sort and organize forms for over 800 Baker Act examinations. The BARC also receives, on average, about 200 petitions and orders for longer term civil commitment each business day. After these more than 1,000 documents are organized, the data are entered into a SQL database. The SQL data entry interface catches some data entry errors (such as warnings to alert if a date of birth entered adds up to an unlikely age), while other data quality issues are addressed en masse by applying data cleaning queries.

FLORIDA MEDICAID DRUG THERAPY MANAGEMENT PROGRAM FOR BEHAVIORAL HEALTH

Program Background

In the early 2000s, the Florida Legislature became increasingly concerned about the rapid rise in expenditures for psychotropic medications in Florida's Medicaid program. Over the 4-year period from 2001 to 2004, these expenditures grew an average of 30% per year and were projected to reach $689 million in state fiscal year 2004–2005; this increase was prior to the implementation of Medicare Part D. While overall Medicaid expenditures on pharmaceuticals were also increasing during this time, the increase in rates for certain classes of psychotropic medications (atypical antipsychotics and antidepressants) was much greater. In response to this growth in expenditures and to concerns about the quality of psychotropic medication prescribing, the 2006 Florida Legislature created the Medicaid Drug Therapy Management Program (MDTMP) for Behavioral Health. The MDTMP is operated by the Florida Mental Health Institute in the College of Behavioral and Community Sciences under contract with the AHCA, the state's Medicaid authority. The goals of the MDTMP, as articulated in Chapter 409.912 (39)(a)(10) Florida Statutes, are to:

- Improve the quality of care and behavioral health drug prescribing practices based on best practices guidelines
- Improve patient adherence to medication plans
- Reduce clinical risk
- Lower prescribed drug costs

The Florida Medicaid Context

In Florida, the AHCA develops and carries out policies related to the Medicaid program. As of 2019, Medicaid serves approximately 4 million people in Florida, with more than half of these children or adolescents 20 years of age or younger.

Most eligible individuals have the choice to enroll in a Medicaid Managed Assistance Plan (MMA); there are currently 12 MMA plans available to Medicaid enrollees. MMA plans are paid prospectively for the care of their enrollees using risk-adjusted capitation rates. In addition, there are a few highly specialized MMA plans.

Purpose of Collaboration, Why It Began, and Who Is Served

Against this background, we describe the processes and sequences used to implement the MDTMP for behavioral health. Our purpose is to describe the MDTMP implemented in the Florida Medicaid system that attempted to integrate a number of different strategies to improve the quality of prescribing practices while employing a variety of tactics designed to modify the practices of selected clinicians.

Process Involved and Implementation

To achieve these program goals, two particular strategies were implemented:

- Evidence-based psychotropic medication guidelines for the treatment of serious mental illnesses in adults and serious emotional disturbances in children were developed.
- Complex care indicators and data filters, indicating practices not supported by evidence, were applied.

How the Collaboration Functions

Based on these guidelines, a series of unusual psychotropic medication indicators (UPMI) were identified and applied as filters to analyze psychotherapeutic pharmacy claims. The analyses identified (1) prescriptions that appeared inconsistent with the guideline recommendations, (2) the patients who filled these prescriptions, (3) the prescribers whose prescriptions frequently triggered the indicators, and (4) the MMA plans to which the patients are enrolled. Educational interventions to improve prescribing practices were developed and implemented for physicians whose prescribing practices fell outside best practices. These clinicians were then targeted for interventions designed to reduce the numbers of their prescriptions that triggered the UPMI. These clinicians were monitored over time for possible follow-up interventions of increasing frequency and intensity. Educational and technological approaches were used to promote best practices, educate consumers, and train prescribers in the adoption of practice guidelines. As part of this approach, a prior authorization review process of selected psychotropic medications was implemented. While this process did not affect a patient's access to psychotropic medications, it improved the quality of psychotropic drug prescribing based on best practice guidelines, improved patient adherence to medication plans, and (most importantly) reduced clinical risk.

Guideline Development and Best Practice Recommendations

The psychotropic medication guidelines are the cornerstone of the program. The first step in implementing this program was to convene a series of panels to formulate specific psychotropic medication recommendations for the treatment of serious mental illnesses in adults and serious emotional disturbances in children. The panels included national experts, representatives from the Departments of Psychiatry of three Florida state universities, psychiatrists in private practice, psychiatrists employed in publicly funded community mental health centers, primary care physicians with an interest in behavioral health, and representatives from the state Medicaid program and other relevant departments of state government. The experts were identified through literature searches and through peer recommendations. The first expert panel for the treatment of adults with schizophrenia, bipolar disorder, and major depressive disorders was convened in 2005 and is updated on a biannual basis. The first expert panel for children with serious emotional disturbances was convened in 2008; the resulting prescription guidelines for attention deficit hyperactivity disorder (ADHD), bipolar disorder, and depression are also updated on a biannual basis.

The updated guidelines reflect the most current medical evidence. Over time some conditions are added to reflect medical advances, and other conditions are eliminated. In addition to the formulation of evidence-based psychotropic treatment guidelines, the expert panels were asked to define several UPMIs derived from the guidelines. The UPMI are data filters that identify prescribing behaviors associated with one or more of the following: (a) are not supported by evidence, (b) produce marginal benefits, and/or (c) increase risks, and therefore should be relatively rare and warrant greater scrutiny. Prescriptions that trigger these indicators represent potential opportunities to improve care.

Significant Changes Since Beginning

There have been a number of recent additions to this program. Among the most recent are

- Women of Reproductive Age with Serious Mental Illness and Co-occurring Substance Use Disorders,

- Monitoring Physical Health and Side-Effects of Psychotherapeutic (Psychotropic) Medications in Adults and Children: An Integrated Approach, and
- Autism Spectrum Disorder and Intellectual Developmental Disorder: Florida Best Practice Psychotropic Medication Recommendations for Target Symptoms in Children and Adolescents.

The current versions of the guidelines, as well as the expert presentations and a wealth of supporting documentation, can be found on our website at: http://floridamedicaidmentalhealth.org.

What Services Are Delivered

As the program evolved, studies were conducted to reflect current concerns on area of interest to the Florida AHCA. For example, in addition to the ongoing monitoring of psychotropic medications, the program analyzed the utilization of long-acting injectable antipsychotics to detect their effectiveness in reducing the utilization of emergency department visits and inpatient hospitalizations, the adverse neonatal outcomes among women of reproductive age with severe mental illness and comorbid opioid use, and the long-term consequences of antipsychotic medication on children under the age of 6 years. The program, in collaboration with AHCA, implemented a prior authorization process for children under the age of 6 years who are prescribed antipsychotic or antidepressant medications.

Analytic Methods

The need to make determinations regarding which clinicians should receive what interventions led to the creation of a database that combined pharmacy claims with several other administrative datasets: enrollment data, eligibility files, professional and institutional claims data, and a national provider database registry and license database. Data are analyzed to identify and provide demographic information on patients whose prescriptions for psychotropic medications triggered one or more clinical indicators. The clinician associated with each of these prescriptions is then recorded. The nature of the clinical indicator triggered for each patient is determined, as well as whether the clinical indicator was the result of the actions of a single prescriber or (when there are duplicate therapies) multiple prescribers. For example, the latter might involve two or more antipsychotic medications prescribed for longer than 60 days when one antipsychotic was written by one prescriber and the other prescription was written by a different prescriber. Individual files were created for each provider whose prescription triggered one or more clinical indicators. Prescribers were grouped into two categories. Those whose population receiving psychotropic medications had a median age of less than 18 years were classified as child prescribers; those with a median age greater than 17 years were categorized as adult prescribers. Finally, adult and child prescribers were ranked separately according to the number of their prescriptions that triggered a clinical indicator, and the percentages of prescriptions that triggered a clinical indicator were calculated for each prescriber. Based on the prescriber's license number, the prescriber was assigned a specialty.

Results

Using the frequency with which each single prescriber triggered a specific clinical indicator, a profile was created and communicated to the prescriber which included a report of their prescribing practices and the patients to whom these medications were prescribed. Three charts per physicians were reviewed in the prescriber's office, followed by an interview to discuss the findings of the chart reviews. Prescribers with a high volume of prescriptions falling outside of evidence-based practice were identified for a peer-to-peer consult. The peer-to-peer consults were strictly voluntary, with the approach intended to be educational rather than punitive. The physicians who performed the peer-to-peer consultations followed a protocol developed by the program and provided a detailed report of the visits. The reports were shared with the physicians. For a period of 1 year, the program followed up with those physicians who participated in the peer-to-peer consults. Over time we observed a reduction in the number of psychotropic medications that triggered consults. Overall, the physicians reviewed were collaborative and appreciative of the opportunity to discuss their prescribing practices with a peer.

Lessons Learned

There were several other well-developed, evidence-based guidelines considered for adoption by Florida, including those of the American Academy of Pediatrics and from the Centers for Disease Control (CDC). We concluded, however, that there were significant benefits to deriving Florida-specific guidelines. (Other states, such as Texas and Ohio, reached the same conclusion.) The inclusion of key expert leaders in this process helped ensure that there were few disagreements about the definition of quality psychotropic medication prescribing practices. While the program began with a lengthy list of UPMIs, the analysis of data quickly led us to focus on antipsychotic polypharmacy and high-dose indicators. This focus on antipsychotic prescribing patterns coincided with the reality that, in Florida, Medicaid expenditures on antipsychotic medications significantly exceeded expenditures on any other class of psychotropic medications.

A large percentage of total psychotropic medication-prescribing activity is concentrated in a relatively small number of prescribers. Potential quality problems associated with psychotropic medication prescribing were even more highly concentrated. This allowed the program to focus its more intensive and expensive interventions on comparatively small groups of providers who were prescribing for adults and children, respectively. Focusing limited resources to achieve optimal quality improvement was helpful to Florida, and we expect it would also be helpful in other states.

PROBLEM-SOLVING COURTS

The drug epidemic that began more than 30 years ago had an extensive effect on the criminal justice system in the United States. Early responses to this epidemic focused on law enforcement and incarceration but had a relatively small impact in reducing drug-related crime (Mitchell, Wilson, Eggers, & MacKenzie, 2012). From these unsuccessful efforts emerged a growing consensus that incarceration without rehabilitation programs is not an effective strategy for interrupting the cycle of drugs and crime. Over the past 20 years, the courts and correctional systems have developed a range of rehabilitation programs intended to reduce recidivism. These include several treatment-based court initiatives, such as problem-solving courts and other specialty court programs (Bureau of Justice Assistance, 2005).

Emergence of Problem-Solving Courts

Problem-solving courts began in the early 1990s in response to significant backlogs and overcrowding in the criminal justice system related to drug offenders and to the ineffectiveness in preventing the rapid cycling and criminalization of this population (Terry, 1999). These alternative programs attempt to address underlying problems of addiction and have incorporated a range of evidence-based treatment principles within the criminal justice system (Hora, Schma, & Rosenthal, 1999). Problem-solving court programs highlight services that provide coordination to facilitate ongoing involvement in community treatment and court supervision.

The Omnibus Crime Control Act passed by Congress in 1994 established the Drug Courts Program Office (DCPO) within the US Department of Justice and provided funding to support the development of drug courts throughout the country. Nearly 500 problem-solving courts were operational by 2001, and, at present, there are more than 3,300 problem-solving courts (National Association of Drug Court Professionals, 2018). Problem-solving courts are now in all 50 states, the District of Columbia, Puerto Rico, and in many other countries.

Problem-solving court programs balance both the community's public safety interests and the rehabilitation needs of participants through collaborative partnerships between criminal justice and treatment systems, as well as a range of ancillary service providers (Longshore, Turner, Wenzel, Morral, Harrell, McBride, Deschenes, & Iguchi, 2001). These programs reduce crime by placing drug-involved offenders in ongoing treatment, which is supervised and monitored by the courts. Compared to traditional criminal courts, problem-solving courts represent a significant departure from adversarial proceedings and operations. Participation is voluntary, although individuals face significant consequences if they do not successfully follow program guidelines. A multidisciplinary team coordinates supervision by the problem-solving court judge and involvement in treatment.

The problem-solving court judges take an active role in monitoring progress in treatment through frequent drug testing and mandatory court appearances. They also encourage participants to stay in treatment through use of a wide range of graduated rewards and sanctions to encourage participant progress (Longshore et al., 2001). Generally, treatment averages about a year, although incentives and sanctions can shorten or lengthen this time. Regular hearings in front of the problem-solving court judge support program guidelines and accountability. A comprehensive set of treatment services are provided by most problem-solving courts and include a phased approach that provides more intensive treatment during the first several months of involvement, followed by less intensive outpatient treatment in later stages of the program (Marlowe, 2010). Treatment typically includes case management, individual and group counseling, random drug testing, peer support groups, mental health services, and a range of other ancillary services tailored to the needs of the individual.

In 2000 and again in 2009, the Conference of Chief Justices (CCJ) and the Conference of State Court Administrators (COSCA) issued joint resolutions concluding that drug courts and other problem-solving courts are the most effective strategy for reducing drug abuse, preventing crime, and restoring families. In recognition of this fact, CCJ and COSCA called on the justice system to extend the reach of problem-solving courts to every citizen in need, and further, to infuse the principles and practices of these proven programs throughout our system of justice. Their conclusions echo more than two decades of rigorous scientific research establishing that drug courts work and that fidelity to the Ten Key Components of the model is essential for achieving the most successful and cost-effective outcomes (see Table 9.2).

Table 9.2 TEN KEY COMPONENTS OF PROBLEM-SOLVING COURTS

Key Component 1 Drug courts integrate alcohol and drug treatment services with justice system case processing.

Key Component 2 Using a nonadversarial approach, prosecution and defense counsel promote public safety while protecting participants' due process rights.

Key Component 3 Eligible participants are identified early and promptly placed in the drug court program.

Key Component 4 Drug courts provide access to a continuum of alcohol, drug, and related treatment and rehabilitation services.

Key Component 5 Abstinence is monitored by frequent alcohol and illicit drug testing.

Key Component 6 A coordinated strategy governs drug court responses to participants' compliance.

Key Component 7 Ongoing judicial interaction with each drug court participant is essential.

Key Component 8 Monitoring and evaluating achievement of program goals is necessary to gauge effectiveness.

Key Component 9 Continuing interdisciplinary education promotes effective drug court planning, implementation, and operations.

Key Component 10 Forging partnerships among drug courts, public agencies, and community-based organizations generates local support and enhances drug court program effectiveness.

National Association of Drug Court Professionals (2004).

Community–University (FMHI) Collaboration

Over the past 15 years, the state of Florida has been very successful in developing and maintaining numerous problem-solving courts. Due to funding cuts within the state on both mental health and substance use funding, courts have forged relationships with university partners. FMHI has had a long history of grant-funded research built on the cooperative relationships with many community-based substance abuse and criminal justice groups and agencies throughout the Tampa Bay area. Within the substance abuse field, these partnerships include professionals at both the administrative level (e.g., CEOs, clinical directors, and program managers) and the clinical level (e.g., counselors, certified addiction professionals, and peer mentors). In the criminal justice setting, partnerships were developed within court administration (deputy directors, drug court program coordinator), the judiciary (drug court judges, drug court specialists), and attorneys (public defender's office, regional counsel, state attorney's office). These relationships often built on one another and have resulted in numerous contract and grant awards.

Purpose of Collaboration

These collaborative relationships were developed over the years and have created partnerships that have resulted in positive systematic changes. These changes have occurred at both the macro (system) and micro (client) levels, resulting in positive impact for both the court system and the community in general. The following is an example of some of the projects funded over the years within Hillsborough County (13th Judicial Court) and describes the functions of these grant-funded programs, their evaluative findings and products disseminated, and the lessons learned from this collaborative effort.

Functions of problem-solving court (who is involved and served). The 13th Judicial Court has collaborated with FMHI on numerous Substance Abuse and Mental Health Service Administration (SAMHSA) grants as a subcontract focusing on the evaluation component. We have been funded by six such SAMHSA drug court grants. FMHI was an integral part of the grant writing process with these grants, totaling $6,925,000; FMHI received $1,996,500 from these six SAMHSA awards. These include the following:

Medication-Assisted Drug Court Treatment (MADCT; 2006–2009). The purpose of this drug court program was to provide a harm reduction–based outpatient treatment option to offenders with opiate use disorder as an alternative to abstinence-based programs or jail or prison, with the ultimate goal of supporting clients in their efforts to achieve sobriety and stability. Successful treatment completion and compliance with drug court requirements allow first-time drug offenders the opportunity to avoid having a felony conviction upon completion of the program.

Marchman Act Drug Court (MADC; 2015–2018). The Marchman Act is a Florida-specific statute allowing families to petition the courts for mandatory assessment and substance abuse treatment. This initiative established the delivery of treatment services from two substance abuse agencies that provided 3–4 months of residential treatment, 2 months of intensive outpatient treatment services, and 2 months of outpatient treatment implementing evidence-based treatment models including *Seeking Safety, Helping Men Recover, Helping Women Recover,* and *Beyond Trauma.*

Veterans Treatment Court (VTC; 2016–2019). This grant program focus is on clients (male and female) who are veterans with substance abuse dependence requiring placement in residential treatment services—and who may also have posttraumatic stress disorder or another substance use or mental health disorder. This court serves defendants with both misdemeanor and felony charges and has both pretrial intervention and post-adjudicatory components. This grant has provided an opportunity for this population to participate in a comprehensive program that integrates court case management with substance abuse treatment and support services. The program provides a multisystem approach to extend residential, intensive outpatient, and recovery support services using evidence-based practices.

Family Dependency Treatment Court (FDTC; 2006–2009, 2012–2015, 2017–2022). FDTCs were established to provide mandated substance abuse treatment services for parents in the child welfare system. FDTC shares key components with drug courts, including a nonadversarial and beneficial experience for those involved. The program was designed to provide a framework to help clients live drug-free and assume the responsibilities of parenthood. Their experience can act as a "springboard" to permanent life changes, specifically those involving alcohol and drug use. A local substance abuse agency, DACCO Behavioral Health, was the contracted treatment provider on the grant and provided 4 months of residential treatment and 3 months of both intensive outpatient treatment services and recovery support using two treatment models.

Effectiveness and Evaluative Findings

Over the past 13 years, there have been numerous benefits as well as challenges that developed with the different problem-solving courts. A brief synopsis of findings from the completed projects is summarized here.

MADCT. Outcomes included high participant graduation rates, significant reductions in criminal justice involvement, substantial decreases in both substance use and mental health symptoms, and more social support and better quality of life following program participation (Moore, Young, Frei, & Barrett, 2012; Young, Moore, French, & Granata, 2012). This MADCT grant resulted in (1) a 69% graduation rate and significant reductions in the arrest rate in the year following program completion, (2) an additional $720,000 for adult drug court treatment in Hillsborough County, (3) positive study outcomes that encouraged the Hillsborough County Judicial Circuit to currently pilot a MAT-centered docket for opioid drug abusers, and (4) dissemination efforts including a dissertation, two evaluation technical reports, and 14 presentations at the local, state, and national level.

MADC. The results of this evaluation indicated that the MADC program is effective in reducing alcohol/drug use and mental health symptoms for those participants who successfully graduated from the MADC program (Moore, Carlson, & Bogovich, 2019). Highlights include (1) high satisfaction rates; (2) decreased rates of substance use; (3) decreased rates of depression, anxiety, overall mental health symptoms, and trauma symptoms; and (4) increased levels of positive social support. Other treatment benefits include decreasing the economic impact of substance abuse on individuals and their families. This grant was just completed in 2020 so dissemination efforts are still in preparation.

FDTC. This study was the first to suggest that an evidence-based FDTC linked to wraparound services both improves reunification rates and reduces foster care readmissions (Chuang, Moore, Barrett, & Young, 2012; Moore, Barrett, & Young, 2012; Moore, Young, Barongi, & Rice, 2015). These two FTDC grants resulted in (1) a 54% family reunification rate compared to 45% in regular dependency court; (2) an additional $1.68 million for FDTC treatment in Hillsborough County;

(3) programmatic enhancements including individualized trauma-informed care, targeted child welfare case management, and expanded wraparound services; and (4) dissemination outreach including three published peer-reviewed articles (with another in preparation), two evaluation technical reports, and 22 presentations at the local, state, and national levels.

Lessons Learned

A necessary element of successful university–community collaborative projects is mutual respect among faculty and community professionals. Both groups have different skills, knowledge, values, responsibilities, and criteria for success and may not be accustomed to sharing control over their projects. Leaders and partners must be willing and able to compromise and find creative solutions. It was in this domain that having leadership at both court and FMHI was especially helpful; each represents the point of view of one profession but simultaneously understands and respects the perspective of the partner.

One challenge that was commonly cited was the limited availability of key stakeholders. Everyone has multiple demands on their time, which makes it challenging to keep communication channels open. Regularly scheduled meetings, particularly in-person discussions, help nurture relationships and provide continuity. Our problem-solving court grantee meetings meet on a monthly basis to stay abreast of needs and identify areas of mutual interest that may yield future research initiatives.

Another valuable aspect of this collaboration has come from embedding students in these projects because these types of assistantships or practicums afford numerous benefits. Students develop an insider's perspective on the mechanics of court structure, nurture relationships with relevant department staff and leadership, and bring those connections back to the university. Students also contribute important knowledge and expertise to resource-constrained projects. Such assistantships enhance student interest in field work and practice-based learning.

Finally, collaborative presentations to community organizations and city officials afford opportunities to disseminate information as well as receive feedback. City officials are more concerned with results and implications than methodology, so it is important for researchers to focus on the "so what?" and the "what now?" They must put findings into the context of community priorities and people's lives.

REFERENCES

Bureau of Justice Assistance (2005). *BJA Drug Court Clearinghouse Project (2005): Summary of drug court activity by state and county (Tech. Rep.)*. Washington, DC: American University. http://www.american.edu/justice/.

Catalano, R., Kessell, E., Christy, A., & Monahan, J. (2005). Involuntary psychiatric examinations for danger to others after the attacks of September 11, 2001. *Psychiatric Services, 56*, 858–862.

Christy, A., Rhode, S., & Jenkins, K., (2020). *The Baker Act: Florida Mental Health Act, Fiscal Year 2018/2019 Annual Report.* https://www.usf.edu/cbcs/baker-act/.

Chuang, E., Moore, K., Barrett, B., & Young, M. S. (2012). Effect of a Family Dependency Treatment Court on child welfare reunification, time to permanency and re-entry rates. *Children and Youth Services Review, 34*(9), 1896–1902.

College of Behavioral and Community Sciences, Louis de la Parte Florida Mental Health Institute (2017). *Annual report.* Tampa, FL: University of South Florida.

Community Mental Health Centers Construction Act (CMHA). (1963, October 31). Public Law 88-164.

Cribb, H. (1966, April 29). Hernando Hospital site said stupid. *Tampa Tribune,* sec. B, p. 2.

Division of Mental Health of the Department of Health and Rehabilitative Services (1969, August 22). *Report prepared for Governor Kirk's meeting* (p. 4). Tampa, Florida.

Florida Administrative Code. (2019). Mental Health Act Regulation: 65E-5. https://www.flrules.org/gateway/chapterhome.asp?chapter=65e-5.

Florida Courts. (2019). Florida trial court statistics. http://trialstats.flcourts.org/.

Florida Department of Children and Families. (1998, Jan.). Ex Parte Order for Involuntary Examination, CF-MH 3001. https://www.myflfamilies.com/service-programs/samh/crisis-services/laws/3001.doc.

Florida Department of Children and Families. (2005a, Feb.). Petition for Involuntary Inpatient Placement, CF-MH 3032). https://www.myflfamilies.com/service-programs/samh/crisis-services/laws/3032.doc.

Florida Department of Children and Families. (2005b, Feb.). Crisis Services Forms. https://www.myflfamilies.com/service-programs/samh/crisis-services/laws/3008.doc.

Florida Department of Children and Families. (2005c, Feb.). Petition for Involuntary Outpatient Services, CF-MH 3130. https://www.myflfamilies.com/service-programs/samh/crisis-services/laws/3130.doc.

Florida Department of Children and Families. (2005d, Feb.). Order for Involuntary Outpatient Services or Continued Involuntary Outpatient Services, CF-MH 3155). https://www.myflfamilies.com/service-programs/samh/crisis-services/laws/3155.doc.

Florida Department of Children and Families. (2006, Sept.). Proposed Individualized Treatment Plan for Involuntary Outpatient Services or Continued Involuntary Outpatient Services, CF-MH 3145). https://www.myflfamilies.com/service-programs/samh/crisis-services/laws/3145.doc.

Florida Department of Children and Families. (2016a, Jun.). Report of Law Enforcement Officer Initiating Involuntary Examination, CF-MH 3052a. https://eds.myflfamilies.com/DCFFormsInternet/Search/OpenDCFForm.aspx?FormId=1062.

Florida Department of Children and Families. (2016b, Jun.). Certificate of Professional Initiating Involuntary Examination, CF-MH 3052b. https://eds.myflfamilies.com/DCFFormsInternet/Search/OpenDCFForm.aspx?FormId=1063.

Florida Department of Children and Families. (2016c, Jun.). Cover Sheet to Department of Children and Families, CF-MH 3118. https://eds.myflfamilies.com/DCFFormsInternet/Search/OpenDCFForm.aspx?FormId=1064.

Florida Department of Children and Families. (2017, Nov.). Taskforce Report on Involuntary Examination of Minors. https://www.myflfamilies.com/service-programs/samh/publications/docs/S17-005766-TASK%20FORCE%20ON%20INVOLUNTARY%20EXAMINATION%20OF%20MINORS.pdf.

Florida Department of Children and Families. (2019, Nov.). Report on Involuntary Examinations of Minors. https://www.myflfamilies.com/service-programs/samh/publications/docs/Report%20on%20Involuntary%20Examination%20of%20Minors.pdf.

Florida Senate. (2004, Nov.). Mental health professionals authorized to initiate involuntary mental health evaluations: Florida Senate interim project report 2005-220. http://archive.flsenate.gov/data/Publications/2005/Senate/reports/interim_reports/pdf/2005-110cf.pdf.

Florida Senate. (2005, Nov.). Clarifying the Baker Act requirements as they relate to children's receiving crisis stabilization units: Florida Senate interim project report 2006-103. http://archive.flsenate.gov/data/Publications/2006/Senate/reports/interim_reports/pdf/2006-103cf.pdf.

Florida Statutes, 120 (Florida Administrative Procedures Act) (2019).

Florida Statutes, 394, Part I (The Baker Act) (2019).

Florida Statutes, 397 (The Marchman Act) (2019).

Hedman L. C., Petrila J., Fisher W. H., Swanson J. W., Dingman D. A., & Burris, S. (2016). State laws on emergency holds for mental health stabilization. *Psychiatric Services, 67*, 529–535.

Hora, P., Schma, W., & Rosenthal, J. (1999). Therapeutic jurisprudence and the drug treatment court movement: Revolutionizing the criminal justice system's response to drug abuse and crime in America. *Notre Dame Law Review, 74*(2), 439–538.

Joint Administrative Procedures Committee. (n.d.). A primer on Florida's Administrative Procedure Act, Joint Administrative Procedures Committee. http://www.japc.state.fl.us/Documents/Publications/PocketGuideFloridaAPA.pdf.

Kessell, E., Catalano, R. A., Christy, A., & Monahan, J. (2006). Rates of unemployment and incidence of police-initiated hospitalization in Florida. *Psychiatric Services, 57*, 1435–1440.

Longshore, D., Turner, S., Wenzel, S., Morral, A., Harrell, A., McBride, D., Deschenes, E., & Iguchi, M. (2001). Drug Courts: A conceptual framework. *Journal of Drug Issues, 31*(1), 7-26.

Marbin, C. A., & Holgren, S. (1995a, May 21). A dangerous Age. *St. Petersburg Times (Florida).* https://advance.lexis.com/api/document?collection=news&id=urn:contentItem:3SNF-5K40-008H-X44X-00000-00&context=1516831.

Marbin, C. A., & Nolgren, S. (1995b, May 22). Locked up voluntarily. *St. Petersburg Times (Florida).* https://advance.lexis.com/api/document?collection=news&id=urn:contentItem:3SNF-5JJ0-008H-X3WN-00000-00&context=1516831.

Marbin, C. A., & Nolgren, S. (1995c, May 23). Tearful and 165 miles from home. *St. Petersburg Times (Florida).* https://advance.lexis.com/api/document?collection=news&id=urn:contentItem:3SNF-5JD0-008H-X3TD-00000-00&context=1516831.

Marbin, C. A., & Nolgren, S. (1995d, May 24). A cure that can kill. *St. Petersburg Times (Florida).* https://advance-lexis-com.ezproxy.lib.usf.edu/api/document?collection=news&id=urn:contentItem:3SNF-5J30-008H-X3MR-00000-00&context=1516831.

Marbin, C. A., & Nolgren, S. (1995e, May 25). One county does it differently. *St. Petersburg Times (Florida)*. https://advance.lexis.com/api/document?collection=ne ws&id=urn:contentItem:3SNF-5HT0-008H-X3F2-00000-00&context=1516831.

Marlowe. D. B. (2010). *Research update on juvenile drug treatment court: Need to know.* Washington, DC: National Association of Drug Court Professionals.

Mitchell, O., Wilson, D. B., Eggers, A., & MacKenzie, D. L. (2012). Assessing the effectiveness of drug courts on recidivism: A meta-analytic review of traditional and non-traditional drug courts. *Journal of Criminal Justice, 40*(1), 60–71.

Moore, K. A., Barrett, B., & Young, M. S. (2012). Six-month behavioral health outcomes of a Family Dependency Treatment Court. *Journal of Public Child Welfare, 6*(3), 313–329.

Moore, K. A., Carlson, M., & Bogovich, S. (2019). *Evaluation of the Marchman Act Drug Court (MADC).* Tampa: University of South Florida, Louis de la Parte Florida Mental Health Institute.

Moore, K. A., Young, M. S., Barongi, M., & Rice, J. (2015). *Evaluation of the Family Dependence Treatment Court (FDTC) Program.* Tampa: University of South Florida, Louis de la Parte Florida Mental Health Institute.

Moore, K. A., Young, M. S., Frei, A. M., & Barrett, B. (2012). *Evaluation of the Medication-Assisted Drug Court Treatment Program.* Tampa: University of South Florida, Louis de la Parte Florida Mental Health Institute.

National Association of Drug Court Professionals (NADCP; 2004). *Defining Drug Courts: The Key Components.* Drug Courts Program Office, Office of Justice Programs, U.S. Department of Justice.

National Association of Drug Court Professionals. (2018). *National Association for Drug Court Professionals fact sheet.* Washington, DC: School of Public Affairs Justice Programs Office, American University.

Policy Surveillance Program. (2016). *Short-term emergency commitment laws.* Philadelphia, PA: Temple University Beasley School of Law. http://lawatlas.org/ datasets/short-term-civil-commitment.

SB12 (2016). Annual, 2016 Regular Session (Florida, 2016). https://www.flsenate.gov/ Session/Bill/2016/0012.

SB1418 (2019). Annual 2019 Regular Session (Florida, 2019). https://www.flsenate.gov/ Session/Bill/2019/01418.

Substance Abuse and Mental Health Services Administration (SAMHSA). (2019). *Civil commitment and the mental health care continuum: Historical trends and principles for law and practice.* Rockville, MD: Substance Abuse and Mental Health Services Administration.

Tampa Times. (1965, Apr. 7). Tampa may get 500-bed state mental hospital. *Tampa Times,* sec. A, p. 6.

Terry, W. C. (1999). Broward County's dedicated drug treatment court: From post adjudication to diversion. In W. C. Terry III (Ed.), *The early drug courts: Case studies in judicial innovation. Drugs, health, and social policy series* (*Vol. 7*) (pp. 77–107). Thousand Oaks, CA: Sage.

Young, M. S., Moore, K. A., French, J., & Granata, S. (2012). *Medication-Assisted Drug Court Treatment Program (MADCT) fidelity to the matrix model.* Tampa: University of South Florida, Louis de la Parte Florida Mental Health Institute.

10

The Development of the Center for Forensic Behavioral Science

A Collaboration Between Forensicare and Swinburne University of Technology

JAMES R. P. OGLOFF ■

Given the nature of forensic psychology and psychology and law, the vast majority of my research and scholarly work has been applied. I have had a long-standing goal to ensure that my research translates into practice and that my work, in turn, is informed by experiences in applied settings. Since 1998, I have held conjoint academic appointments and leadership positions in public forensic or correctional services. Despite the inevitable tensions that exist between "the ivory tower" and "the front line," I believe that my work has been greatly enriched by the need to balance the demands of both employment cultures. At the same time that I have held professorial appointments, I was the inaugural Director of Mental Health Services for British Columbia Corrections (1998–2001) and then Director, and later Executive Director, of Psychological Services and Research for the Victorian Institute of Forensic Mental Health (known as Forensicare) in Victoria, Australia (2001–present). Research and scholarly writing typically affords free rein in considering novel ideas and ideal circumstances. Indeed, academic freedom and the freedom of enquiry are cornerstones of academia. By contrast, prison and mental health services must be highly agile and pragmatic, dealing with a host of ongoing challenges and crisis situations (for instance, at the time of writing, we are navigating the plethora of challenges in the face of the COVID-19 pandemic). These schisms in philosophy, approach, and, indeed, epistemology, require ongoing thought. It has been my experience, inevitably, that simultaneously considering research and applied services leads both to more valid research and to service development that is informed by the rigors of evidence-based practice.

Drawing on my experience, this chapter describes the collaboration between the Victorian Institute of Forensic Mental Health, known as Forensicare, and Swinburne University of Technology (SUT) in Melbourne, Australia. Established in 2006, the Center for Forensic Behavioral Science (CFBS) serves as both the research and training arm of Forensicare, the statewide forensic mental health service in Victoria, Australia, and a research center within SUT. Victoria is Australia's smallest mainland state, with a size roughly equivalent to Oregon and a population of approximately 6.5 million, similar to Indiana. Most (77%) of the population of Victoria reside in the capital city, Melbourne, which is a multicultural metropolis of more than 5 million people, with more than one-third of the people speaking languages other than English at home. The collaboration that has developed between the forensic service and the university is unique in Australia.

VICTORIAN INSTITUTE OF FORENSIC MENTAL HEALTH (FORENSICARE)

As the statewide forensic mental health service, Forensicare was initially established in the state's mental health act in 1997 (Mental Health [Victorian Institute of Forensic Mental Health] Act, 1997). Forensicare is a statutory agency responsible for the provision of adult forensic mental health services in Victoria (Forensicare, 2019). Forensicare employs almost 800 staff members, 85% of whom are clinicians (444 nurses [of whom 389 are registered psychiatric nurses]), 71 medical practitioners (39 forensic psychiatrists, 31 psychiatric residents, and 1 medical officer), 73 psychologists (a blend of clinical, forensic, and clinical/forensic psychologists), 33 social workers, 28 occupational therapists, 1 art therapist, and 1 social welfare officer. The organization also has placements across all of the disciplines.

It is governed by a Board of up to nine directors who are appointed by the Governor in Council for 3-year terms on the recommendation of the Minister for Mental Health. The Board is responsible for establishing the strategic direction and governance framework of the organization and monitoring compliance. As Figure 10.1 depicts, Forensicare provides clinical services across three directorates: Prison Mental Health Service, Thomas Embling Hospital, and the Community Forensic Mental Health Service. The Prison Mental Health Services provide forensic mental health services across all of the public and private prisons in Victoria. Mental health nurses screen all incoming prisoners for mental illness upon admission, and a variety of services are then provided across the system. These include "bed-based" services as well as "outpatient" services within the prisons. The bed-based services include a 16-bed Acute Assessment Unit at the Melbourne Assessment Prison, a 75-bed service (including acute, rehabilitation, and personality disorder units) at Ravenhall Prison, a 30-bed recovery and rehabilitation unit at Port Phillip Prison, and a 44-bed mental health unit at the Dame Phyllis Frost Center—the state's prison for women. Outpatient services, provided to prisoners residing in units other than the bed-based mental health

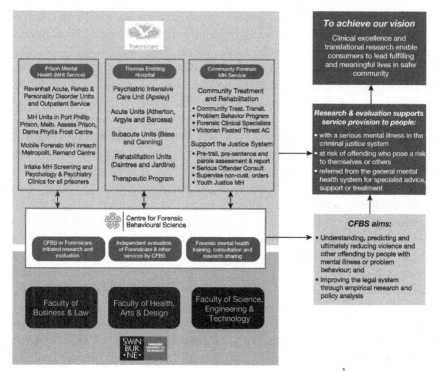

Figure 10.1 Clinical services provided by Forensicare and the interface with the Center for Forensic Behavioural Science (CFBS).

units, include psychiatry and psychology sessions across most prisons, as well as the Mobile Forensic Mental Health Service at the Metropolitan Remand Center. There are also 100 outpatient spaces available at Ravenhall Prison.

The Thomas Embling Hospital includes 136 beds configured across seven units in a high-security precinct and low-security unit. The units comprise an 8-bed psychiatric intensive care unit for prisoners requiring involuntary psychiatric care, two 17-bed male acute units, one 12-bed female acute unit, one 22-bed long-stay male unit, a 24-bed mixed-gender subacute unit, and a 20-bed mixed-gender rehabilitation unit. Male and female patients in the 16-bed low-security unit are accommodated in independent living unit flats outside of the secure perimeter but still confined within a wire mesh fence. The hospital provides the panoply of forensic mental health assessment and intervention services for the state and includes prisoners transferred from prison for involuntary psychiatric care as well as forensic psychiatric patients (those found unfit to stand trial or not guilty because of mental impairment—equivalent to incompetent to stand trial and not guilty by reason of insanity in the United States).

The Community Forensic Mental Health Service (CFMHS) includes a community treatment and transition team to help integrate prisoners with mental illnesses back into the community and a similar service for forensic patients transitioning back into the community after discharge from the Thomas Embling Hospital. In addition, it operates a Problem Behavior Program (Warren, MacKenzie, Mullen, & Ogloff, 2005) that provides assessment and/or treatment to people in the criminal justice system—or at risk of entering the criminal justice system—as a result of their "problem behaviors" (e.g., sexual offending, stalking, threatening, violence). Clients are drawn from both the mental health system and the criminal justice system. The CFMHS also operates the Victoria Fixated Threat Assessment Center in partnership with Victoria Police to help identify and manage fixated threateners and lone actor grievance-fueled violence perpetrators. The CFMHS also coordinates a clinical forensic specialist service for statewide area mental health services for adults and youth. Finally, the CFMHS conducts the pretrial and presentence assessments for the courts as well as assessments for the parole board.

In addition to providing specialist clinical services through an inpatient and community program, Forensicare is mandated (under the Mental Health Act, 2014) to provide research, training, and professional education. Specifically, the statutory functions and powers of Forensicare include the mandate "to conduct research in the fields of forensic mental health, forensic health, forensic behavioural science and associated fields" and to "promote continuous improvements and innovations in the provision of forensic mental health and related services in Victoria" (Mental Health Act, 2014, s. 330(g) & s. 330(h)). Forensicare's mandate to conduct research is quite unique among forensic mental health services in Australia. All too often, a tension exists between research and practice in clinical services, and forensic mental health services are typically no different. Within Forensicare, however, there is a critical nexus between science and practice, with each informing the other to ensure excellence and evidence-based practice in our service. Ongoing research in forensic behavioral science and forensic mental health is critical owing to the highly specialized nature of the field and the rapidly emerging knowledge in the field.

SWINBURNE UNIVERSITY OF TECHNOLOGY

SUT was founded as a technical college in 1908. It gained university status in 1992 (Swinburne University of Technology Act, 1992). The university has more than 23,000 students, including almost 4,000 graduate students. SUT is primarily located on a campus in Melbourne, but has satellite campuses in the state and one in Sarawak, Malaysia. The university is organized into three faculties: Business and Law; Health, Arts, and Design; and Science, Engineering, and Technology. The CFBS is located in the School of Health Sciences within the Faculty of Health, Arts, and Design.

PURPOSE OF THE COLLABORATION

Despite the legislative mandate that Forensicare conduct research, Forensicare has traditionally received very little government funding to further this responsibility.

From its inception, Forensicare has worked with a range of universities to develop a research capacity in forensic mental health and related fields. The relationships have ensured that Forensicare attracts academics and research funding to undertake research relevant to Forensicare's clinical work. The CFBS operates under the auspices of SUT in collaboration with Forensicare. The CFBS serves as the research arm of Forensicare, conducting independent research and facilitating the research enterprises of Forensicare and as a research and teaching center in the Faculty of Health, Arts, and Design at SUT. SUT was keen to have the CFBS join it because the university had established an undergraduate program in psychology and forensic science in 2011 (the only such program in Australia), and the addition of the CFBS was complementary since it provided for the establishment of graduate training in forensic behavioral science (forensic mental health, forensic psychology) and enhanced the university's reputation in those fields.

THE ESTABLISHMENT OF THE CENTER FOR FORENSIC BEHAVIORAL SCIENCE

Professor Paul Mullen, a prominent forensic psychiatrist and prolific academic, was appointed Foundation Professor of Forensic Psychiatry at Mont Park Hospital (psychiatric hospital that included a forensic mental health service) and at Monash University in 1992 (Ogloff, 2010). At the time of his appointment, forensic psychiatry had a low profile in Victoria and patients were held in old facilities that were not built for this purpose—many dating from the Victorian era. There was very little research being undertaken in forensic mental health, with legal processes and clinical practices left wanting by international standards. Forensicare was established in 1997, to provide forensic mental health services in Victoria, and the Minister for Health appointed Professor Mullen as the inaugural Clinical Director. Mr. Michael Burt, a former social worker and head of the prisoner health service, was appointed the inaugural chief executive officer. They shared a vision to establish Forensicare as a center for excellence in forensic mental health and they set out to do so. In 1998, Monash University created the Doctor of Psychology (clinical) course that included a specialization in clinical forensic psychology. A Chair in Clinical Forensic Psychology was established between Forensicare and Monash University, and, in 2000, I was appointed to that chair. In that same year, Forensicare opened a purpose-built 100-bed secure forensic psychiatric hospital, the Thomas Embling Hospital.

In 2004, the CEO of Forensicare and the Dean of the Faculty of Medicine, Nursing, and Health Sciences at Monash University commissioned an independent consultation to review the research undertaken in the forensic mental health area and the relationship between Forensicare and Monash University. The key recommendation was to create a department in the University to promote further development of the areas of forensic mental health and forensic behavioral science. At the time, however, Monash University was moving away from establishing small departments in favor of larger schools. In this context, the decision was made to establish a center rather than a department to fill the gaps identified in the review. The CFBS was approved by the Faculty of Medicine, Nursing, and Health Sciences at Monash University in 2005 and commenced in January 2006. I was appointed as the Director of the CFBS, a position which I still hold.

Forensic behavioral science concerns the study of factors that underlie offending and human behavior in the legal system. Forensic behavioral scientists are interested in understanding how individual characteristics interact with the environment to produce criminal behavior and what might be done to prevent such behavior in the future. Forensic behavioral science informs practice in the field of forensic mental health including the disciplines of psychology, psychiatry, mental health nursing, health sciences, social work, and occupational therapy. These professionals are responsible for the assessment and treatment of those who are or have the propensity to become mentally disordered and whose behavior has led or could lead to offending. More broadly, forensic behavioral science concerns the way in which offenders are identified and managed by law enforcement, courts, and criminal justice systems. It includes both clinical and experimental approaches to understanding the legal system.

The CFBS was established in 2006 and grew to include academic staff in forensic psychiatry, forensic psychology, forensic mental health nursing, and law. At the outset, the CFBS had three staff members: the Director, Deputy Director, and Professor Mullen. Two part-time senior lecturers in forensic psychiatry were appointed, and, in 2008, a fulltime senior lectureship in clinical forensic psychology was established and Dr. (now Professor) Michael Daffern was appointed. We also had a Professor of Forensic Mental Health Nursing Practice join the CFBS part-time in 2008 and then move to a full-time position in 2011. Unfortunately, when she retired in 2012, the position was not replaced. Professor Mullen retired from his role as Clinical Director of Forensicare and, in 2009, was appointed Professor Emeritus. A professor of forensic psychiatry/assistant clinical director (research) for Forensicare position was created and filled. The CFBS began to enjoy a growing national and international reputation for excellence in research and training.

Unfortunately, the School of Psychology and Psychiatry at Monash University, in which the CFBS was situated, was dismantled, along with a number of changes in philosophy and direction. As such, the decision was made for the CFBS, and the relationship with Forensicare, to seek arrangements with an alternative university. In January 2014, the CFBS relocated from Monash University to SUT. The move enabled the CFBS and the Forensicare research program to thrive and for SUT to expand its profile in forensic psychology and forensic mental health, adding a research and postgraduate training capacity.

THE CURRENT ORGANIZATION, GOVERNANCE, AND STAFFING OF THE CFBS

As noted previously, the CFBS operates both as a research center within the Faculty of Health, Arts, and Design at SUT and as the research and training arm of Forensicare. The CFBS is comprised of researchers with backgrounds in clinical and forensic psychology, forensic psychiatry, forensic mental health nursing, criminology, and law. As set out in Figure 10.1, the CFBS aims include (1) understanding, predicting, and ultimately reducing violence and other offending by people with mental illness or problem behavior and (2) improving the legal system through empirical research and policy analysis.

Figure 10.2 depicts the organizational structure of the CFBS and the relationship to Swinburne University and Forensicare. Legally, a Master Collaboration Agreement (MCA) has been established between SUT and Forensicare. The MCA provides for the governance of the CFBS, the conduct of research, intellectual property, and further opportunities between SUT and Forensicare. In addition, it contains standard terms that address matters of confidentiality and publication, use of logos, warranties, insurance and indemnification, default and termination, and dispute resolution.

Operation and governance of the CFBS is primarily the responsibility of SUT. The Director reports to the Dean of Health Sciences in the Faculty of Health,

Forensicare and CFBS organisational arrangements

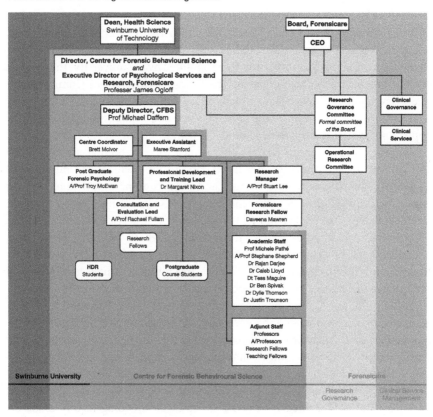

Figure 10.2 Organizational structure of the Center for Forensic Behavioral Science (CFBS) and the relationship to Swinburne University and Forensicare.

Arts, and Design. The Director also has an informal reporting relationship to the Dean of Research for the Faculty through to the Deputy Vice-Chancellor (equivalent to a vice-president) of Research and Enterprise for the University. The University reviews the CFBS annually, as part of its review of all research centers in the University. The Director also holds a concurrent appointment as Executive Director of Research and Psychological Services for Forensicare and, in that role, reports to the Chief Executive Officer. He also attends and provides support the Forensicare Swinburne Research Governance Committee, a Committee of the Forensicare Board.

There are two standing committees that manage and monitor the CFBS: the Joint Management Committee and the Forensicare-Swinburne Research Governance Committee. There is a Joint Management Committee with equal membership from SUT (Dean, Faculty Manager, Professor) and Forensicare (CEO, Executive Director of Clinical Services, Chief Financial Officer), as well as the Director, Deputy Director, and Research Center Coordinator of the CFBS. The purpose and function of the Joint Management Committee is to coordinate, monitor, and report on the activities between Swinburne and Forensicare under this MCA and to explore opportunities to collaborate and strengthen the relationship between the University and Forensicare.

The Forensicare-Swinburne Research Governance Committee is a committee of the Forensicare Board and includes the CEO of Forensicare; two Forensicare board members; the Dean of Health Sciences; Dean of Research for the Faculty of Health, Arts, and Design; and a professor appointed by the university. The Director of the CFBS is an ex-officio member. The Research Governance Committee is a senior-level, joint governance forum providing both parties with the ability to effectively monitor and evaluate the research value and future strategic partnership opportunities arising from their joint investment in the CFBS.

The progress and success of the CFBS is measured by both academic metrics and clinical service priorities. Academic monitoring includes the number and quality of publications, research grants, and other funding awarded; impact and engagement; and student numbers and completions. The clinical service priorities are included to ensure that the CFBS satisfies the strategic research needs for Forensicare, including the need for translational research and service evaluation. There is a goal, as well, to involve Forensicare staff members and consumers in research and to help ensure that the Forensicare culture continues to reinforce the importance of evidence-based practice and continuing clinical excellence.

Funding for the CFBS comes from four sources: SUT, Forensicare, income generated from research, and income generated from training. SUT provides approximately two-thirds of the ongoing funding for the operation of the Center. The University receives income from the more than 40 doctoral and 300 postgraduate students enrolled in the CFBS. The University also receives research infrastructure and overhead income from grants and research and training contracts. Funding from SUT primarily covers salaries of the ongoing faculty members, the Center Coordinator, equipment, services, rent, and utilities for the CFBS. Forensicare contributes funds toward rent, as well as salaries of the Director,

Executive Assistant to the Director, nursing, and psychiatry academics. In addition, Forensicare funds a full-time Research Manager, as depicted in the organizational chart. Most of the research undertaken in the CFBS is funded by either competitive grants or contract research/evaluation. Finally, the CFBS engages in a range of contract professional development training for justice and human service agencies as well as nongovernmental organizations. Importantly, although members of the CFBS staff are paid for—variously—by SUT, Forensicare, or jointly, the staff work together cooperatively to meet the goals of the CFBS.

As set out in Figure 10.2, the CFBS is led by the Director and Deputy Director, both of whom are professors. The Director has a conjoint appointment as Executive Director of Psychological Services and Research with Forensicare, while the Deputy Director holds a substantive appointment with SUT and has a part-time clinical appointment as Principal Consultant Psychologist with Forensicare. Administrative assistance is provided by a Center Coordinator and an Executive Assistant to the Director. The Center Coordinator provides administrative oversight, including financial, human resources, and facilities. The CFBS includes four leadership positions: Consultation and Evaluation Lead, Professional Development and Training Lead, the Post Graduate Forensic Psychology Lead, and the Forensicare Research Manager. Each of these staff members oversees a particular area of work undertaken by the CFBS, as outlined here.

CFBS staff members include 14 academic staff members: three professors, three associate professors, five senior lecturers, two lecturers, and the Forensicare Research Manager (who holds an adjunct associate professor appointment). There are nine postdoctoral research fellows who work across the research areas. The CFBS also relies on a large number of adjunct clinical, research, and teaching staff members (17 clinical associates, 8 teaching fellows, 11 research fellows, 1 senior research fellow, 4 adjunct associate professors, and 4 adjunct professors). At the time of writing, the CFBS has 42 doctoral students (17 PhD students and 25 completing the Doctor of Psychology, with a Clinical and Forensic Psychology specialization degree). We also have 320 enrollments in our post graduate courses in Forensic Behavioral Science.

We have also benefitted greatly from a relatively regular flow of visiting academics who have spent time with us in the CFBS. We have capitalized on the SUT visiting professor program and have hosted some academics on sabbatical. This regular flow of people with new ideas and perspectives has been helpful to staff and students alike.

The CFBS holds an annual planning day and regular staff meetings. Of course, smaller groups of members meet on particular projects. Early on, the Director served as the supervisor and mentor for each staff member. These tasks were then shared with the Deputy Director. More recently, as we have had added capacity at the associate professor level, we have shared these duties more broadly. We have mentoring sessions and processes for early-career researchers and graduate students.

Although Forensicare is our only formal partner, the CFBS enjoys close working relationships with a number of other government agencies and organizations. For example, the CFBS has engaged in a variety of research and evaluation projects with the Department of Justice and Community Safety (DJCS). These projects have included contract evaluation and research, externally funded collaborations, researcher-initiated projects, and doctoral student research projects. These projects have been conducted across a range of DJCS areas, including Corrections Victoria, Victoria Police, Youth Justice, and Court Services Victoria. We have also engaged in a number of projects nationally and internationally with different organizations.

THE OPERATION OF THE CFBS

The CFBS has a vision to be Australasia's leading center for excellence in the areas of forensic mental health and forensic behavioral science research, teaching, and practice development. It is envisaged that the CFBS will evolve and strengthen the field of forensic behavioral science and forensic mental health, both in Australia and internationally. A key focus of the CFBS is to transfer academic and clinical excellence into practice in the health, community services, and criminal justice sectors.

To achieve its vision, the CFBS engages in (1) conducting original research in topics pertaining to forensic mental health and forensic behavioral science, (2) providing first-rate postgraduate training in graduate programs in forensic mental health and forensic behavioral science that attract increasing numbers of high-caliber students, (3) providing continuing professional development workshops to enhance the knowledge and skill base of the work force, and (4) providing expert consultancy and training in mental health, law, and related sectors.

Research

The CFBS has achieved a great deal of success in meetings its aims. Our researchers represent many disciplines and publish their work in leading national and international journals. The research conducted in the CFBS falls into seven themes: (1) aggression and violence; (2) complex criminal behavior; (3) culture, psychology, and law; (4) forensic mental health; (5) psychology and legal processes; (6) rehabilitation, reintegration, and offender management; and (7) young people, offending, and victimization. Each theme is facilitated by one or two academic staff members.

Most of the academic staff members are prolific researchers, and the CFBS has produced almost 800 peer-reviewed articles, more than 100 book chapters, and nine books in the 14 years since its inception. In addition, more than 70 industry reports have been published. Staff have had good success securing competitive research grant funding from the Australian Institute of Criminology, Australian Research Council, the National Health and Medical Research Council, and other local and national funding schemes (e.g., Law Institute of Victoria). In accordance with our aims and goals, all research undertaken in the CFBS is applied and has implications for clinical practice and the justice system. Staff members have made many unique research contributions to the field that have resulted in changes to practice in Australia and internationally. Staff members have developed and validated several empirically supported risk assessment measures that are used nationally and internationally (e.g., Dynamic Appraisal of Situational Aggression; Ogloff & Daffern, 2006; Stalking Risk Profile; MacKenzie et al., 2009; and the Victoria Police Screening Assessment for Family Violence Risk; McEwan, Shea, & Ogloff, 2019). In addition to advances made in risk assessment, CFBS staff are leading figures in developing theoretical and empirical approaches to more effectively intervene with offenders.

Teaching

The CFBS operates two successful streams of graduate programs: forensic behavioral science and forensic psychology. The graduate program in forensic behavioral science offers a range of courses in forensic mental health (see Box 10.1) and forensic behavioral science that lead to seven possible degrees: (1) Graduate Certificate in Forensic Behavioral Science, (2) Graduate Diploma in Forensic

---

Box 10.1

CENTER FOR FORENSIC BEHAVIORAL SCIENCE (CFBS) COURSE OFFERINGS IN FORENSIC BEHAVIORAL SCIENCES

Core Skills in Forensic Practice
  Fundamentals of Criminal Law Process
  Working in Corrections and Youth Justice
  Principles of Violence Risk Assessment and Management
  Advanced Violence Risk Assessment and Management
  Mental Disorder and Offending
  Working with Difficult Personalities in the Forensic Context
  Substance Misuse and Offending
  Trauma and Offending
  Development, Developmental Disability and Offending
  Problem Behaviours 1 (violence, threats, intimate partner violence and
    fire-setting)
  Problem Behaviours 2 (stalking, abnormal complaining, and harmful sexual
    behaviours towards children and adults)
  Forensic Mental Health Nursing (restricted to nurses)
  Forensic Mental Health Nursing Practice (restricted to nurses)
  Psychiatry in Forensic Contexts (restricted to psychiatrists)

Behavioral Science, (3) Masters of Forensic Behavioral Science, (4) Graduate Certificate in Forensic Mental Health Nursing, (5) Graduate Diploma in Forensic Mental Health Nursing, (6) Graduate Certificate in Forensic Psychiatry, and (7) Graduate Certificate in Specialist Forensic Assessment and Risk Management.

These are full fee-paying programs. More than 320 students enroll in the courses annually. Students are drawn from all of the mental health disciplines (i.e., nursing, psychology, psychiatry, social work, occupational therapy) as well as those who work in the broader sector. While most students are from Victoria, approximately one-third are from interstate, with growing numbers of overseas students. The courses are all conducted online, with a possible field school occurring once each semester.

The graduate program in forensic psychology provides training accredited by the Australian Psychology Accreditation Council leading to either a Graduate Diploma in Forensic Psychology or a Doctor of Psychology (Clinical and Forensic Psychology). The Graduate Diploma in Forensic Psychology is a part-time 2-year program that enables registered psychologists with endorsement in another area (e.g., clinical psychology, clinical neuropsychology) to undertake coursework and supervised clinical forensic placements to satisfy the requirements for endorsement as a forensic psychologist. The Doctor of Psychology (Clinical and Forensic Psychology) is a 4- to 5-year program that provides clinical, research, and supervised placement training leading to endorsement as both a clinical psychologist and forensic psychologist. This program is unique in Australia. The intake for these courses combined is 8–9 students per year, with approximately 25–30 students in residence at any given time.

Consultation and Evaluation

The CFBS provides expert consultancy, service evaluation, and research consultancies to industry. These consultancies not only provide a bridge between the university and the sector, but also generate income for the CFBS that is used for research and operational costs. Consultancies have covered a range of topics and have been conducted for a range of agencies, including, for example, program evaluations for forensic services, service evaluations, validation of assessment measures, and evaluation of training initiatives. The research and evaluation component of the CFBS's work has grown steadily over time; in 2020, we established a Consultation and Evaluation Lead and appointed Associate Professor Rachael Fullam to that position (Figure 10.2).

Professional Development and Training

As part of its mandate to engage with industry and provide professional education, the CFBS holds monthly research colloquia to which clinicians and researchers are invited. We hold an annual public lecture where a prominent person is the invited speaker. We also host a biennial international conference. The CFBS also provides a range of professional development training, either under contract to agencies (e.g., corrections, human services, police) or organized by the CFBS for paying participants. We are also working with Forensicare to coordinate and deliver all external training offerings. In 2020, we established the position of Professional Development and Training Lead and appointed Dr. Margaret Nixon to that role (Figure 10.2).

ACCOMPLISHMENTS

Given the vision and aims of the CFBS, our most significant contributions have been the influence our work has had on policy, practice, and law. Our work is regularly cited by Australian courts, law reform commissions, royal commissions, and government reports. Many staff members sit on advisory groups and boards within government and nongovernmental organizations. Research conducted in the CFBS has led to significant developments in forensic mental health and forensic psychology. Center staff have developed and validated several empirically supported risk assessment measures that are used internationally. Primary among these is the Dynamic Appraisal of Situational Aggression (DASA; Ogloff & Daffern, 2006) that evaluates the risk of inpatient aggression among psychiatric patients. There is also a youth version for youth justice and youth mental health services. The DASA has been researched extensively internationally and has been recognized by the National Institute for Clinical Excellence in the National Health Service, United Kingdom, as best practice for assessing and managing inpatient aggression (National Institute for Health and Care Excellence, 2015).

The accomplishments of the CFBS have also been realized in awards and other distinctions accumulated by our staff. As already noted, CFBS staff members are prolific researchers, and their work has had significant impact across policy- and decision-making in Australia and beyond. Two staff members have won Fulbright Fellowships. The Director and Deputy Director have both received distinguished contribution awards from professional associations, and staff members have similarly received early distinguished career awards from national and international associations (e.g., American Psychology Law Society, Australian Psychological Society, and International Association of Forensic Mental Health). Several staff members have also received teaching and research awards from SUT (and Monash University previously). I have recently been appointed as University Distinguished Professor, the highest honor for an academic in the university.

Members of staff have also held leadership positions in professional associations. For example, two members have served as President of the Australian and New Zealand Association of Psychiatry, Psychology, and Law, and two have served as Chair of the College of Forensic Psychology for the Australian Psychological Society. One is a board member of the International Association of Forensic Mental Health Services. Two members are Fellows of the Australian Psychological Society, and the Director is also a fellow of the American Psychological Association,

Canadian Psychological Association, and the International Association of Applied Psychology. I was appointed a Member of the Order of Australia (AM), part of the Australia honors system, for "significant service to education and to the law as a forensic psychologist, as an academic, researcher and practitioner" (see https://honours.pmc.gov.au/honours/awards/1150891).

Several members have extensive editorial board experience with journals. This includes an editorship (*International Journal of Forensic Mental Health* [IJFMH]), associate editorships (*BMC Medical Education, Criminal Justice and Behavior* [CJB], *International Journal of Offender Therapy and Comparative Criminology*, IJFMH, *Law and Human Behavior*), and editorial boards (e.g., currently *Behavioral Sciences and the Law*; CJB; IJFMH; *Journal of Psychiatry and Psychology*; *Journal of Threat Assessment and Management*; *Law and Human Behavior*; *Psychiatry, Psychology, and Law*).

Perhaps most importantly, the legacy of the CFBS is reflected in the many doctoral students and other postgraduate students we have trained. Of the more than 60 doctoral students and postdoctoral research fellows who have completed their training with us, many hold academic positions and senior clinical leadership positions. Several have won dissertation and early-career awards, and a large percentage of our students are awarded competitive scholarships that fund their education. A number of graduates have also entered public service, working in research and policy positions.

EXPERIENCES AND LESSONS LEARNED

In the 15 years of operation of the CFBS, we have experienced a number of challenges and enjoyed many opportunities. On reflection, the CFBS has grown and prospered to an extent well beyond what we initially anticipated. Along the way, we have also made mistakes and had to change pathways. Initially, a considerable amount of effort and diplomacy was required to establish the CFBS. The necessary processes in a university to establish an academic unit are typically onerous, and that certainly was the case for us. Even with the support of the Forensicare leadership group, we needed to obtain the approval of the Forensicare Board. The initial period of operation of the CFBS, while growing gradually, was quite positive with a number of early successes.

One of the most significant challenges we have faced, though, was the need to relocate from our original university at the end of 2013. As noted earlier, the CFBS was housed in the School of Psychiatry and Psychology at Monash University. Due to a number of changes in personnel, the school was dismantled and the direction of the new School of Psychological Sciences was focused on biological psychology. Vacancies in the CFBS were not being replaced. The decision was made to move from Monash University to another academic home. It was fortuitous that SUT had developed an undergraduate forensic science and psychology program and planned to establish a school of health sciences. Negotiations were undertaken between SUT and Forensicare for the relocation of the CFBS to SUT. The then-Chief Executive Officer of Forensicare, Mr. Tom Dalton, and the Forensicare Board maintained their support for the CFBS throughout. In January 2014, we transitioned from one university to the other. Given that the CFBS was located at a Forensicare site, we did not move—but we did change the sign outside of the Paul Mullen Center and the CFBS! Rather, the responsibility for the administration of the CFBS moved. A huge effort was undertaken to establish the postgraduate programs outlines in Figure 10.2 and discussed earlier at SUT. Six years later, the move has been incredibly positive for the CFBS, Forensicare, and SUT. The CFBS has grown considerably, and the relationship between CFBS and SUT has expanded.

Beyond these two issues, a number of broader considerations have led to the success of the CFBS and may serve as an indication of elements of successful academic–clinical service collaborations. These considerations fall into six categories that will be discussed next: vision and perseverance; staff and culture; space, equipment, and facilities; facilitating collaboration; budget and finance; and being responsive and flexible.

Vision and Perseverance

Like any successful venture, the starting point requires the capacity to envision what can be. This involves the ability to see opportunity and have the foresight to capitalize on it. In the case of the CFBS, we were fortunate that the first Clinical Director of Forensicare, Professor Paul Mullen, and the inaugural CEO, Mr. Michael Burt, shared a vision of developing excellence in forensic mental health. I was recruited to assist in helping to fulfill the vision. Early on, we realized that it would not be possible to obtain adequate government funding to establish a meaningful research and training program without the collaboration of a university. To this end, since both Professor Mullen and I held academic chairs in a university, we were able to get the strong support of the Head of Psychiatry and the Dean of the faculty. As noted, this led to an external review, to which we of course contributed. The alignment of these individuals—and their support—allowed us to establish the CFBS. Initially the Center only included the two of us. We quickly set out to build a vision for the CFBS and to recruit.

The long-term opportunities for the CFBS were abundant, but it took many years to develop the Center. At any point, it would have been easy to stop expending the energy to develop and grow the Center. There were certainly no readily identifiable personal benefits for our work. This is where perseverance comes in. The CFBS has now survived three Forensicare CEOs and clinical directors, four Forensicare Board Chairs, three Monash Deans, two Swinburne Deans and another two Executive Deans/Pro-Vice Chancellors, four heads of school, and more than 20 Forensicare board members and other leaders. All throughout, we have had to continue to "tell our story" and convince those who led us about the value of the CFBS.

Staff and Culture

To establish a viable and strong team, our internal focus has been on the identification and development of staff. Our goal has been to foster a collegial and
supportive culture, but one that challenges staff and allows staff members to fulfill
their own goals while supporting the vision of the CFBS. A significant challenge
for us has been the location of the CFBS in Australia—which is far from both
North America and Europe, where most of the international work in forensic
mental health is done. As such, we have employed a two-pronged strategy that
has involved both training and developing local people and selectively recruiting
international ones.

The focus on developing a collegial culture has involved supporting staff and
ensuring a good fit among colleagues. When I was a young academic on a hiring
committee during my first academic job, after we interviewed a particularly promising candidate, showed her out, and closed the door, the most senior member of
the committee said, "Well, would you have lunch with her for the rest of your
life?" I laughed, thinking that he was joking. To my surprise, however, he said
that academic positions were unlike any other jobs—particularly in contemporary times—since people stayed for many years, often for life. In employing people
thereafter, I have thought almost as much about collegiality and fit as I have about
academic prowess. The latter can be developed but the former, in my experience,
are characteristics that are generally intractable.

In addition to considerations regarding collegiality and fit, our strategy has
been to identify staff to play one (or more) of a host of roles necessary to run a
successful Center. To this end, we value staff for the role that they play and recognize that every member has different strengths—all of which must be valued.
To be successful in the academic/clinical space we occupy, it has been very important to ensure that most staff members have both clinical experience and academic prowess. Given the role we play in teaching—and the animosity that some
researchers have for such work—we have ensured that we have a strong compli-
ment of good teachers and teaching leaders. Beyond actual roles, we have been
fortunate that so many staff members have helped build a collegial culture by
having social events—both formal and informal. This "professional socialization"
helps ensure that it is enjoyable to come to work each day (although that has now
become digital contact since I am finalizing this chapter during the time of the
COVID-19 workplace restrictions that have us working from home).

The value of professional support staff cannot be overstated. I have benefitted
from an extraordinary executive assistant, Maree Stanford, who has been with us
since the very beginning (and before). Similarly, the appointment of our Research
Center Coordinator, Mr. Brett McIvor, when we relocated to SUT in 2014 was
much welcome; he has served us so well over the years.

As we have reached a critical mass, the culture among the postdoctoral
fellows and graduate students has also become a significant feature of the CFBS.
Particularly in the modern era that makes it easy to work away from the Center,
it is important that postdoctoral fellows and students enjoy being onsite and

working together—even though the interests and research that they undertake can be very different from one another.

Space, Equipment, and Facilities

When it was established, the CFBS was housed in the administration building at Forensicare's Thomas Embling Hospital. We had no purpose-built or configured space, and staff were distributed around the organization and the university. This was a decided disadvantage, as the arrangement did not facilitate the informal and chance discussions that are so vital to both relationship-building and opportunities for collaboration. So, having dedicated space where research staff can work together along with postdoctoral fellows and students is important in the successful establishment and development of a center.

In 2009, the CFBS co-located with the Community Forensic Mental Health Service of Forensicare, in a building that was most fittingly named the Paul Mullen Center. For the first time, this enabled us to configure and renovate space that met the Center's needs. While the offices and research space were enclosed in dedicated space, the CFBS shared the facilities, amenities, meeting rooms, and seminar room with Forensicare. Being co-located with Forensicare's clinical services had decided advantages. It allowed for easy access to clinical populations, clinical records, and, most importantly, clinical staff. Being in shared space also ensured that the CFBS was very much part of Forensicare.

Unfortunately, by 2016, both the Forensicare Community Forensic Mental Health Service and the CFBS had grown, and the growth could not be accommodated within the Paul Mullen Center. Unsurprisingly, as is the case with universities worldwide, there was no way to adequately accommodate the CFBS within the University. For all of the reasons mentioned earlier regarding the benefits of being located at (or close to) Forensicare, a site was located close to Forensicare sites. The CFBS is now housed in a commercial building some 1.5 miles from the Thomas Embling Hospital and 2 miles from the Community Forensic Mental Health Service. We occupy more than 8,000 square feet, with a large meeting space in which we hold workshops and other training sessions, a seminar room that can accommodate postgraduate teaching and other meetings, a kitchen, break-out space, adequate office space for all academic staff and postdoctoral fellows, and open plan workstations for graduate students and research assistants. At the time of this writing, plans are afoot for expanding the Thomas Embling Hospital, which would include expanded space on-site for the CFBS. It is too early to tell if these plans will eventuate, but the CFBS staff and our partners at Forensicare are keen to see the Center returned to hospital site.

Although there are certain advantages to being co-located with clinical services, there are also disadvantages to being away from the university. The adage "out of sight, out of mind" is all too true. As such, we strategically take steps to build and foster connections with SUT. These include having an office in the psychology department at the University to be used by staff members when we are working there or attending meetings. We make a point of hosting senior staff from the University at the CFBS to ensure they are acquainted with us and the work that we do. As noted earlier, we host our colloquium series at the CFBS and invite both clinicians from Forensicare and academic staff and students from SUT. We also encourage academic staff, particularly junior ones, to visit the university and get to know—and to be known by—staff members there. Also, graduate students attend classes on campus, but all of the postgraduate clinical forensic psychology and forensic behavioral science classes are taught on-site at the CFBS.

Facilitating Collaboration

There is no doubt that a successful collaboration is the most essential element in successful university and public behavioral health organization collaboration. From my experience—as a lawyer, psychologist, academic, clinician, and administrator—interagency and interdisciplinary collaborations may happen by chance, but they are not developed and grown by chance. Thus, a significant part of my time as director, and that of the staff and students, is spent fostering and building collaborative relationships. Also, as a public statewide mental health service, the CFBS has had to be responsive to government priorities, realized both through Forensicare and by virtue of our work more broadly in the public service. We have done this by ensuring that our work is shared with senior public servants and government ministers. (In Australia, ministers serve in the cabinet of the government are and equivalent to secretaries in the United States.) We are decidedly apolitical—to ensure that we are seen as independent at time of government change. While there can be a short-term benefit to being allied with the government of the day, this does not bode well when there is a change in government. The work of the CFBS has been valued by successive governments of different persuasions over many years.

In this chapter, I have detailed the relationship that has been cemented between SUT and Forensicare. It is difficult enough to foster a successful relationship with one organization, let alone two. Moreover, the culture of universities is very different from forensic mental health services. Thus, it is essential to continually foster the relationship with both entities—and between the entities as well. One of the challenges is that the cycle of personnel transition between the two organizations varies. For example, the Forensicare Board Chair and members are appointed for a period of 3 years. The CEO serves a term between 3 and 5 years and cannot serve more than two terms. By contrast, the Dean of Health Sciences has a 5-year appointment. Similarly, other senior staff members' terms vary between the two organizations. What this effectively means is that it is rare that more than 1 year passes before there is some leadership transition. As such, there is an ongoing need to educate people about the CFBS and to essentially convince them of its value. It is inevitable that periods of time occur where one organization or the other is more or less favorably disposed to the Center.

Our approach to the partnership has been to be completely transparent in our dealings with both entities. Also, as noted elsewhere in this section, we constantly strive to ensure that the work of the CFBS fits into the strategic goals of the organizations. For example, SUT has a "Swinburne 2025" strategic plan that promotes research that is "innovative, collaborative, relevant and internationally recognized" and "focus[es] on outcomes and impact through close engagement with industry and the broader community" (https://www.swinburne.edu.au/about/strategy-initiatives/2025-strategic-plan/). Similarly, Forensicare's Strategic Plan notes that "we lead research on mental illness and offending to inform policy and program advocacy, including early intervention, prevention and community safety" (https://www.forensicare.vic.gov.au/now-available-strategic-plan-201819-202021/). Thus, as part of our work, we aim for our research to satisfy both the University's goals, as well as those of Forensicare. Similarly, the training conducted in the CFBS—both formal university programs and professional development offerings—needs to meet the education and professional development goals of the organizations.

The final strategy that we have found useful is to ensure that senior staff at the University meet and become familiar with their counterparts at Forensicare. These personal relationships help ensure that the parties get to know each other and realize that while they come from very different workplace perspectives, they can share common goals in the operation of the CFBS. Given the staggered transition of personnel over time, ensuring that there are always some leaders with knowledge and a corporate memory of the collaboration also helps to indoctrinate new members into the collaboration group.

Although Forensicare is the only formal partner of the CFBS, as noted earlier, we regularly engage in research and complete consultations with a range of organizations, including the justice, human service, and education departments in Victoria and nationally. This variety enriches both our research and work, but it also helps ensure the financial viability and relevance of the Center.

Budget and Finance

The university and forensic mental health service collaboration has a healthy tension in the financial support of the CFBS. Our strategy all along has been to ensure that, at worst, the CFBS breaks even financially; ideally, it realizes a return on investment for the host organizations. As such, we have ensured that we have diverse income streams: income from student fees, contract research and consultation, and competitive grant funding. We are now at a point in our development that the CFBS is cost neutral or returns a small investment to the University. While financial gain is important, the ancillary benefits that the CFBS brings to both SUT and Forensicare are also important. For Forensicare, as noted at the outset, the Mental Health Act (2014) requires that it conducts research and provides education and training. Thus, the goal is to ensure that the CFBS can do this in a cost-effective manner. Also the CFBS enhances the reputation of Forensicare and has served as an attractive feature in the recruitment of medical staff and other senior clinical staff members who are aware of the Center and may have an interest in an affiliation with us.

Apart from student tuition and fees, which goes directly to the university, most of the income of the CFBS comes from contract research and evaluation projects and competitive grant funding. These income streams fund the research fellows and research assistants who work in the CFBS, as well as some of the staff members, such as the Consultation and Evaluation Lead. We have worked diligently to grow this aspect of our work to help ensure our long-term financial viability. We have also been growing the value of our contract training work. To date, this has largely entailed having contracts with state departments and non-governmental organizations to provide training to their staff members regarding matters within our expertise. We are working with Forensicare to develop external training workshops that we can offer to individuals and organizations for a fee. Some of this training will be delivered online.

Given our financial dependence on SUT and Forensicare, it is important to demonstrate our value to them. As noted earlier, this is done in a number of ways, including being diligent to ensure that the work we undertake fits within the strategic directions being undertaken by the host organizations. We are also flexible and responsive to changing government and societal priorities to ensure that our work remains relevant—and provides opportunities to capitalize on the priorities that are fashionable within our areas of interest and expertise.

Being Responsive and Flexible

Although the work of the CFBS falls well within the forensic mental health–forensic behavioral science interface, we have had to be flexible as well. There are two reasons to remain responsive and flexible. The first is to remain relevant in times of change, and the second is to ensure that we can capitalize on current funding priorities and opportunities. For me, as a long-standing researcher, I have ongoing research interests that I have pursued over decades now. The same is true with other academic staff members in the CFBS. Over time, though, we have had to pivot and tailor our interests and sometimes pursue different areas of work. For example, since its inception, the work of the CFBS has expanded to include arson—largely in the face of the growing problem of arsonists in the hot dry Australian summer that has contributed to large-scale destruction (Ducat & Ogloff, 2011; Stanley, March, Ogloff, & Thompson, 2020). Similarly, we have developed a program of research on inpatient aggression, family violence, victimization, young offenders, and cultural aspects of forensic mental health—all in response to growing and changing needs. Most recently, in the face of COVID-19, we are establishing research to investigate the reliability, acceptability, applicability, and integrity of forensic tele-health assessments for courts and judicial tribunals. We have recently undertaken a survey of forensic psychologists and psychiatrists as we begin to explore this area.

THE FUTURE

Just as it was not possible to see the future in 2006, when the CFBS was established, it is impossible to know what the future for the Center holds at this time. As always, though, a number of challenges—and opportunities—are on the horizon. COVID-19 has already had a devastating effect on the economy and has resulted in operational changes to both SUT and Forensicare. In particular, the University Sector in Australia has been detrimentally affected given its reliance on international students as well as local enrollments. There are projections that Australia's research capacity will be greatly affected by this crisis (see https://www.science.org.au/sites/default/files/rrif-covid19-research-workforce.pdf).   Already, SUT staff members have been asked to accept voluntary pay reductions and to donate to the university. It is still early days, so it is not possible to foresee the long-term effects of the pandemic on the long-term prospects of the CFBS. Indeed, the Vice-Chancellor and President of SUT who supported the CFBS's relocation is retiring and will be replaced in a few months. Other changes in SUT's senior leadership team have recently occurred. These changes, as noted earlier in this chapter, necessitate us to be proactive in "telling out story" and convincing the leadership group of the importance of the Center going forward.

Contrasting with the uncertainties arising from the pandemic, there are many positive developments on the horizon that should bode well for the continued success of the CFBS. Forensicare has undergone significant growth and transformative change in the past 5 years, growing by 40%. They have transitioned to a new Chief Executive Officer, Dr. Margaret Grigg, who has long-standing expertise in mental health, administration, and the public service. Similarly, the Forensic Board is comprised of highly experienced individuals with very strong backgrounds in a number of areas, led by Mr. Ken Lay AO, the Lieutenant Governor of Victoria and a former Chief Commissioner of Victoria Police. The CFBS continues to be supported and valued by the leadership team. As noted, plans are afoot to redevelop the Thomas Embling Hospital and to develop purpose built space for the CFBS at the hospital site.

A particularly positive development is the Victorian Government's establishment in 2019 of the Royal Commission into Victoria's Mental Health System. (A royal commission is a major formal public inquiry into a defined issue. Royal Commissions occur in countries in the Commonwealth and have considerable powers, including subpoenaing witnesses, taking evidence under oath, and requesting documents.) It was established to investigate deficiencies in the state's mental health system and the broader prevalence of mental illnesses and suicides in the state. There are four eminent commissioners and an Expert Advisory Group with eight members, including the Director of the CFBS. The commission published and delivered its interim report in late 2019 (Royal Commission into Victoria's Mental Health System, 2019) and will finish its work by the end of October 2020. The interim report recommended the establishment of the "Victorian Collaborative Center for Mental Health and Wellbeing" which will "bring people with lived experience together with researchers and experts in multidisciplinary

clinical and non-clinical care to develop and provide adult mental health services, conduct research and disseminate knowledge with the aim of delivering the
best possible outcomes for people living with mental illness. The centre will work
within a network of partners including service and research organisations in rural
and regional areas" (Royal Commission into Victoria's Mental Health System,
2019, p. 391). The report cites the CFBS as an example of a collaborative research
center operated cooperatively by a health service and university. As noted earlier,
with the establishment of the Victorian Collaborative Center for Mental Health
and Wellbeing comes an expectation that there will be a number of partners, including research organizations, to help realize the Collaborative Center's vision.
We are working to position the CFBS as one of those partners.

The ongoing success of the CFBS will continue to depend on recruiting a steady
stream of highly capable doctoral students and research fellows. Similarly, the success of the CFBS is owed to its academic staff, and we must continue to ensure
that we recruit and retain highly qualified staff. Also, with the ageing CFBS leadership, succession planning must figure prominently in the Center's future plans.
Rejuvenation is important for the long-term viability of any organization (Boal &
Hooijberg, 2000).

CONCLUSION

The development of fruitful collaborations between universities and public behavioral health organizations in justice contexts is challenging, but doing so effectively can be rewarding and can provide benefit to the host organizations. In this
chapter, I have traced the development of the CFBS, a research and training center
within SUT, and the training and research arm of the statewide forensic mental
health service in Victoria, Australia—Forensicare. The CFBS began to satisfy
Forensicare's statutory obligations to provide research, training, and professional
education in forensic mental health and forensic behavioral science. This requirement has been realized by partnering with SUT to further its goal of leading the
forensic mental health and forensic psychology training and research space in
Australia and New Zealand.

Over 15 years, the CFBS has grown and developed. The current organization
and governance of the Center satisfies the requirements of both the University
and forensic service. The CFBS has established an international profile in research
and is perhaps best known for that work. It provides a unique suite of university programs to educate forensic psychologists, forensic psychiatrists, forensic
mental health nurses, and other forensic mental health professionals, and others
who work at the intersection of behavioral science and mental health and the
law. The CFBS also provides expert consultancy, service evaluation, and research
consultancies. This work has ensured that the CFBS remains financially viable and
current. Finally, the work of the CFBS includes the delivery of professional development and training.

The organizational structure, staffing, and governance have evolved to support and monitor the ongoing work of the CFBS. Both SUT and Forensicare have governance requirements that the CFBS must satisfy. In addition, there are two levels of joint governance and monitoring committees (at the executive and board levels) to help ensure that the CFBS meets the needs of both host organizations.

The work of the CFBS has had considerable impact by influencing policy, clinical practice, and law. Staff members and students are well-regarded, have held leadership positions in professional organizations, and have been the recipients of many awards and honors. Many staff are also active in editorial positions in journals in our field.

On reflection, the challenges—and successes—of the CFBS fall into six categories. I discuss each of these as examples of matters that need to be considered by those engaged in developing collaborations between universities and public behavioral health organizations in justice contexts. These include the need for vision and perseverance; fostering staff and culture; securing adequate space, equipment, and facilities; facilitating collaboration; and being responsive and flexible given changing times and priorities.

Working in these environments, and leading the CFBS through its development and ongoing evolution, have been incredibly gratifying. While the level of commitment and the amount of work required by such an undertaking is extraordinary, it has been entirely worthwhile (though not without some disappointments along the way). It is my hope that the description of our journey, along with the learning and experiences along the way, may be of some benefit to others who work in such collaborative settings—or who aspire to develop and facilitate them.

REFERENCES

Boal, K. B., & Hooijberg, R. (2000). Strategic leadership research: Moving on. *Leadership Quarterly, 11*(4), 515–549.

Ducat, L., & Ogloff, J. R. P. (2011). Understanding and preventing bushfire-setting: A psychological perspective. *Psychiatry, Psychology and Law, 18*, 341–356

Forensicare. (2019). *Annual report 2018–2019.* Melbourne, Australia: Victorian Institute of Forensic Mental Health. https://www.forensicare.vic.gov.au/wp-content/uploads/2019/10/201910-FC-Annual-Report-2018-19-FINAL-WEB.pdf

MacKenzie, R. D., McEwan, T. E., Pathé, M. T., James, D. V., Ogloff, J. R. P., & Mullen, P. E. (2009). *Stalking risk profile: Guidelines for the assessment and management of stalkers.* Melbourne: StalkInc & Centre for Forensic Behavioural Science, Monash University.

McEwan, T. E., Shea, D. E., & Ogloff, J. R. P. (2019). The development of the VP-SAFvR: An actuarial instrument for police triage of Australian family violence reports. *Criminal Justice and Behavior, 46*, 590–607. doi:10.1177/0093854818806031

Mental Health Act. (2014). Victorian Acts. https://www.legislation.vic.gov.au/in-force/acts/mental-health-act-2014/022

Mental Health (Victorian Institute of Forensic Mental Health) Act. (1997). Victorian Acts. https://www.legislation.vic.gov.au/as-made/acts/mental-health-victorian-institute-forensic-mental-health-act-1997

National Institute for Health Care and Excellence. (2015). Violence and aggression: short-term management in mental health, health and community settings. NICE guideline [NG10]. https://www.nice.org.uk/guidance/ng10

Ogloff, J. R. P. (2010). Evolution of forensic mental health services in Victoria. *Criminal Behaviour and Mental Health, 20*, 232–241. https://doi.org/10.1002/cbm.773

Ogloff, J. R. P., & Daffern, M. (2006). The Dynamic Appraisal of Situational Aggression: An instrument to assess risk for imminent aggression in psychiatric inpatients. *Behavioral Sciences and the Law, 24*, 799–813.

Royal Commission into Victoria's Mental Health System. (2019). Interim report. Melbourne, Australia: Author. https://rcvmhs.vic.gov.au/interim-report

Stanley, J., March, A., Ogloff, J. R. P., & Thompson, J. (2020). *Feeling the heat: The prevention of wildfire: International perspectives on the prevention of wildfire ignition.* Wilmington, DE: Vernon Press.

Swinburne University of Technology Act. (1992). Victorian Acts. https://www.legislation.vic.gov.au/repealed-revoked/acts/swinburne-university-technology-act-1992/045

Warren, L. J., MacKenzie, R., Mullen, P. E., & Ogloff, J. R. P. (2005). The problem behaviour model: The development of a stalkers clinic and a threateners clinic. *Behavioral Sciences and the Law, 23*, 387–397.

11

Collaboration Between Universities and Public Behavioral Health Organizations

Analysis and Discussion

KIRK HEILBRUN, CHRISTY GIALLELLA,
H. JEAN WRIGHT II, DAVID DEMATTEO, PATRICIA GRIFFIN,
BENJAMIN LOCKLAIR, DAVID AYERS, ALISHA DESAI,
AND VICTORIA PIETRUSZKA ■

The various chapters in this book have described different projects in which there has been collaboration between a university and a public behavioral health organization. There have been some variations in how these collaborations have worked. One chapter, for instance, addressed the process of a collaboration between different units within a university (Chapter 7), while another offered a description of the development of relevant services for the courts but without contracting with a specific agency (Chapter 4). Even considering such differences, however, the descriptions of these various collaborations provide important common ground. Before considering how such collaborations begin and are sustained and the lessons they can provide to any considering beginning such collaborations, however, we should make several points. The sampled collaborations are not necessarily representative of such projects more broadly. These particular examples were selected because of their longevity and success. They probably have much to teach us about the successful implementation, operation, and sustainability of such collaborations—but possibly less about the range of challenges that can limit the success of collaborations between university and public behavioral health personnel. With those caveats in mind, let us turn to some of the common aspects of successful collaborations of this kind and the lessons to be drawn from them.

BEGINNING COLLABORATIONS

One of the important common elements of these collaborations concerns their leadership. Successful operations requires leadership on both the academic and public organization sides of the collaboration. Most of these successful projects are led on the university side by individuals who spent a number of years in leading the collaboration. They were not necessarily very senior in their field, particularly when they first became involved with the collaboration. But they were sufficiently established in their respective areas to have the skills and competence to address certain needs in the public behavioral health sphere and to lead others in this process. Equally important, they were *perceived* as skilled and competent. These leaders, without exception, were also interested in *applying their skills to solving problems in the public domain*. Without such interest, it seems unlikely that many of these collaborations would have been as successful or durable as they have been.

Other aspects of these partnerships are more varied. In some, the "client" is the public behavioral health organization receiving services in the form of consultation, training, and continuing education. In others, the services are provided to individuals who are part of the clientele served by the agency (e.g., hospitalized individuals, justice-involved adolescents, mental health professionals). Selecting the projects that are most similar in purpose, scope, and services to a collaboration being considered is one useful approach to drawing guidance from these chapters.

The financial support provided in the course of any collaboration is a necessary part of the decision to commit time and resources over a lengthy period. There are at least three models for developing such support. One involves a contractual agreement between university and public organization partners: services in designated areas and with specified deliverables are provided in exchange for a specified total cost. As may be seen in the preceding chapters, such contracts are typically renewable annually and can be discontinued at the discretion of either partner. A second model involves an agreement to jointly pursue extramural funding from granting agencies and foundations. A third approach involves the development of services (often in training or continuing education) that are provided on a fee-for-service basis to others outside the university or the public organization. Revenue from such services to third parties can be used to offset the cost of other services provided as part of the collaboration. Several of the collaborations described in this book used more than one of these funding models (see, e.g., Chapters 5, 9, and 10). There was also a frequent emphasis on the need for creativity in addressing funding challenges. Funding was never seen as stable or straightforward; several projects indicated that available funding from some sources had actually decreased over the years. This created challenges. Successful projects were able to resolve or at least manage these challenges using creativity and a shared interest in continuing the collaboration.

SUSTAINING COLLABORATIONS

Each of these collaborations occurred over multiyear periods. There were several common elements apparently involved in sustaining them. There must be an accurate perception of initial need addressed through a collaboration that provides genuine value to both parties. The importance of stable leadership on at least one side of the collaboration is also clear. For different reasons, the collaborations in the preceding chapters were often associated with having a single leader, or small group of leaders, on the university side and more rapidly changing leadership on the public organization side. This meant that there had to be constant attention paid to the nature of the services and the value they provided. New leaders on the public organization side were not necessarily convinced (in the same way that the original leaders had been) that this collaboration was justifiable. Third, the importance of mutual respect and effective communication was evident. The ongoing challenges in areas such as funding, shifting priorities, and changing personnel were approached as problems to be solved through mutual commitment and creativity.

Measuring service effectiveness involves important recurring questions that were answered somewhat differently across projects. Some were quite detailed in specifying goals and measuring deliverables, leading to a fairly straightforward discussion as part of the annual partnership renewal question. Others included services that were broader and less easily measured but still considered under the broader "perception of value" rubric. Some of the partnerships focused generally on certain priorities and services over the years. Others expanded considerably, or otherwise adjusted their goals and deliverables, according to changing priorities of the agency. Partnerships that featured "consultation" prominently among these priorities were likely to require more flexibility and seemed harder to measure— beyond the more general perception that a service was valuable. Those including education such as continuing education (CE) presentations or other specific services were more likely to include greater detail in the measurement of deliverables. But considering that contractual arrangements were typically renewable annually, there was always attention to whether the services provided during the past year had been in the expected quantity and value to help decide whether the contract should be renewed. Since these chapters describe collaborations that were annually renewed over multiyear periods, it is useful to consider how this effectiveness question was addressed (and how this varied) across projects.

One exception to the "annual renewal" aspect of the collaboration may be seen in Chapter 10. This Australian collaboration—currently between Forensicare and the Swinburne University of Technology—differs in some important respects from those described in the other chapters. It is the only featured collaboration outside the United States; this clearly allows us to consider less information but raises intriguing questions about how these collaborations function globally. Second, it is considerably larger than any of the other collaborations described in this book. This illustrates how this kind of academic–public behavioral health partnership can be implemented and sustained on a larger scale. But the size of the collaboration has resulted from sustained growth using a multiple funding strategies, demonstrating the scope of what can be achieved with the combination of leadership, vision, and mutual needs.

LESSONS LEARNED

What can be learned from the limited literature on the topic of university–public behavioral health collaborations? What can the descriptions of the nine successful projects in this book add to our knowledge? In this section we turn to the topic of what these projects, viewed in the context of the larger literature, can teach us. Such collaborations have the potential to provide great value—relevant and effective services that would not otherwise be available—in an era in which public funding for such services is often limited or variable. But such partnerships are also challenging to develop, operate, and sustain. In this section, we discuss the lessons that chapter contributors have offered from their particular projects. These lessons have been organized into the following domains: starting a collaboration, planning, working together, training, consultation, financial considerations, personnel, and research. Those interested in a specific kind of project will find it valuable to consider these "lessons learned" in conjunction with the chapter(s) describing collaborations that are most similar to their own partnerships.

Starting a Collaboration

One consistent aspect of these collaborations is the presence of a university leader with expertise and interest in the general domain area. This is not necessarily generalizable to other university–public behavioral health collaborations. It is striking, though, that each of these projects has been led by a single leader or a small group of individuals over a period of years. But having expertise and an interest in public application is only part of the story. There must be initial contact between the agency leader(s) and the university. In some instances (e.g., Massachusetts; see Chapter 3), the vision for the collaboration began with the public organization, which made the first contact with those who would become university partners in the collaboration. So the second component contributing to start-up involves awareness of relevant needs and available resources.

Since a number of these projects began at a time when such knowledge was disseminated differently—when books, journal articles, and professional presentations were not supplemented by websites, powerful search engines, blog posts, and social media—such awareness is developed differently circa 2020 than it was even a decade ago. Those with the requisite expertise and interest are now easier to locate. This might make it easier to take the initial steps in starting a collaboration. But it does *not* necessarily mean that such collaborations are also easier to operate or sustain (Worden, McLean, & Bonner, 2014). As we discuss in the remainder of this section, there are aspects of the collaborative work that might even be more difficult when "personal contact" includes e-mailing, texting, and remote conferencing. These tools undoubtedly make communication easier and contact more convenient. Whether they can fully substitute for other aspects of in-person contact remains to be seen. This is worth considering as we discuss other lessons in this chapter.

Planning

Successful collaborations are facilitated by careful planning. In this section, we discuss the aggregated suggestions from earlier chapters on planning for successful collaboration. These include clarifying project goals, controlling the volume of referrals, collecting data, tailoring services to context, anticipating how demand for services may change over time, the importance of flexibility, piloting and field testing, understanding the broader context, and initiative sustainability.

Clarity is needed in the project's mission, goals, and deliverables. Some of these collaborations are very focused and lend themselves to a high degree of specificity in developing the mission, setting the goals, and agreeing on products or outcomes to be delivered. Clear expectations regarding expected deliverables has been cited as a "key ingredient" for successful collaborations (Nilson, Jewell, Camman, Appell, & Wormith, 2014; Rudes, Viglione, Lerch, Porter, & Taxman, 2014). One good example appears in Chapter 3, in which the University of Massachusetts Medical School and the Massachusetts Department of Mental Health collaborated to develop a training and certification program for professionals providing forensic mental health assessments for the legal system. This involved developing training materials, a means of evaluating proficiency, a process for supervision, and other products or services that could be measured—along with outcomes of the training and certification. Another example can be seen in Chapter 7, in which one particular university psychologist with expertise in threat assessment worked with other units within the university to develop an approach to assessing and intervening with individuals who appeared to present a risk of harm to others. Both of these collaborations involved a fairly high degree of specificity and the collection of relevant data, which could be used as part of ongoing discussion of project continuation and modification.

By contrast, collaborations that were broader and included a number of domains in which advice and consultation were integral were still able to describe their mission and goals but in a way that was necessarily less specific and harder to quantify. Good examples of this can be seen in the collaborations in Virginia (Chapter 2) and Ohio (Chapter 5). Clarity in specifying mission, goals, and deliverables is seen as desirable. But the extent of that clarity depends on the nature of the articulated need and the approach to addressing that need. Furthermore, whether a collaboration is highly focused depends on the priorities of both partners, but particularly those of the public organization. Attempting to specify and even quantify less tangible services such as consultation can be labor-intensive. Satisfying this priority under those circumstances would come at a cost, which would have to be considered as part of the overall collaboration.

Control the volume of referrals and be clear on requests and products. One project (Chapter 4) involved the provision of services (psychological evaluations of legally involved individuals) to the courts in Texas. Although payment for such services was "contracted" in the sense that each evaluation was provided for an identified, capped fee, there was no easy way to control the number of referrals within this arrangement. Since the cost per evaluation was less than courts would pay to private evaluators, the university clinic received more requests for evaluation than they could provide using their initial resources. Their advice under such circumstances is to anticipate the possibility of significant growth and to use market influence to limit the number of referrals. In other words, establish a price per evaluation that is not so low as to create a compelling financial incentive to provide a larger number of referrals than can be covered—unless the project is prepared to grow considerably.

Collect ongoing data. Each of these collaborations described some form of data gathering. These data were retained and used for purposes such as modifying services, improving products, enhancing trust and communication, and discussing contract renewal. The *nature* of these data—whether quantitative or qualitative—followed from the specificity of the services and products and from the preferences of the collaborative partners. But there is little doubt that the ongoing collection of data in some form serves multiple purposes for successful collaborations. Data collection is one of the most basic elements of such partnerships across public health, business, medicine, and the social sciences (Childs & Potter, 2014). Depending on the level of interest in research, some collaborations include conducting research that goes well beyond that directly applicable to policy and clinical practice (see, e.g., Chapter 10). But most of the collaborations focus on collecting data that are directly relevant to these applied areas.

Fit services to context. There is an implicit assumption across all projects that the services offered will address the identified need. This is probably so obvious that none of the chapter authors discuss it much. But what becomes apparent when reviewing all chapters is the wide range of services that *could* have been provided. Offering clinical consultation and supervision worked very well in certain contexts (see Chapter 6, describing the relationship between the University of California-Davis School of Medicine and the California Department of Mental Health), but would not have been nearly as useful in addressing the broader system-level goals in another (Ohio, for instance; see Chapter 5). Perhaps one ingredient of a successful collaboration is the careful consideration of the match between the identified needs of the public organization and the skills and interests of the university partners. When there is not a good fit, this is likely to create potentially insurmountable problems for the success of the collaboration. But as collaborations expand, additional team members can be brought on to share in the leadership and service provision. This allows the provision of relevant services without relying only on the skills of current team members.

Anticipate that demand for services may grow. Almost without exception, the projects described in these chapters grew considerably over the years. This involved both delivering more of the same kinds of services (see Chapter 4, for example, describing the expansion of services providing psychological evaluations to the courts) as well as services in additional domains. The oldest project described in these chapters—the Institute of Law, Psychiatry, and Public Policy—has grown from an initial collaboration providing training to a multidomain partnership that now includes training, consultation, research, and leadership (see Chapter 2). Those entering into initial collaborations should thus consider the possibility that successful partnership in one area may lead to a request for expanded services in the same area, or in additional areas. It is likely that there is a substantial demand for services that *could* be met through such collaborations, although it is currently not (Rojek, Smith, & Alpert, 2012).

Flexibility is important. The more expansive the goals of the collaboration, the more important it is be flexible. One project (Chapter 8) underscores the value of incorporating such flexibility into the design and implementation of major system reform, drawing on rapid-cycle improvement theory and methodology. The value of flexibility and creativity in other areas, such as collaborations and funding, may also be seen in Chapter 5. In some respects, this may seem inconsistent with an earlier lesson involving clarity in the project's mission, goals, and deliverables. We reconcile the two as follows: while clarity and specificity are important, particularly in the early stages of a collaboration, it is not possible to anticipate all challenges that may arise in the attempt to achieve broader system-level change. Accordingly, it is particularly important to retain some flexibility in how such challenges are addressed while still working closely with all parties involved in the collaboration. This is clearly illustrated by the structural changes in the collaboration described in Chapter 10, in which the university partner changed because of various lost or diminished resources available from the first partner.

Use piloting and field testing. One of the important tools in such collaborations is small-scale testing of measures and procedures that may eventually be implemented on a much larger basis. This is used in developing a test or measure for research purposes; it is even more valuable when trying to implement a procedure to be applied in the field. Good examples of this kind of piloting are seen in Chapter 5 (with Sequential Intercept Model mapping workshops) and Chapter 8 (using Graduated Response as an alternative approach in working with juveniles on probation). When research is "difficult to use," this is an important barrier to applying it in many contexts (Pesta, Blomberg, Ramos, & Ranson, 2019). This can be addressed by smaller scale pilot data collection, allowing the usefulness of the research to be appraised and modified as needed.

Understand services in broader contexts. Collaborations should be informed by relevant scientific evidence and standards of practice. One particular advantage of a collaboration of this kind is the knowledge that should be contributed by university partners regarding scientific evidence and practice standards—knowledge that can then be contextualized using the policy and practice expertise of the public agency partners. Providing the broader scientific and professional standards context should be expected from university partners in such a collaboration, either from immediate knowledge or background research.

Create a sustainability plan. Some collaborations are intended to be time-limited (Worden et al., 2014). When the original goals are achieved, there may be less need for continued collaboration. But it may also be that the collaboration shifts from one domain to another after the original goals are achieved. When the initial goal involves collaboration that is intended to transition into having agency staff provide the agreed-upon services, this may require additional planning to ensure that the work is successfully transitioned while the changes are sustained. See Chapter 8 for an example.

Working Together

One of the key ingredients of these collaborations involves how the partners develop a complementary working style. This is one of the features of such collaborations that has existing empirical support, particularly when such partnerships are "truly collaborative" (Sullivan, Willie, & Fisher, 2013). The importance of the relationship between collaborating partners is often stressed (see, e.g., Burkhardt et al., 2017; Pesta et al., 2019; Rudes et al., 2014; Sullivan et al., 2013). Some of the chapters (e.g., Chapters 5 and 8) focus on this in detail. This section addresses several lessons that are either cited explicitly by chapter authors or inferred from their discussion.

Obtain buy-in from leadership in both academic and agency partners. This can be interpreted in two ways. It is important to have a strong commitment from those who are leading the collaboration, both from the academic and public agency sides. But these individuals typically report to other leaders, whether within the university (e.g., department heads, deans, provosts) or the public organization (e.g., division head, agency head, commissioner). These "other" leaders should be aware of the project, its needs and distinctive aspects, and its strengths. In times of uncertainty created by turnover or when there is financial stress, it can be invaluable to have the support of senior leaders on both sides. In some instances, it may be advantageous to have some senior leaders with an appointment to both academic and agency organizations (see Chapter 10, for example).

Cite advantages to both partners. A distinctive aspect of academic–public agency collaboration involves the advantages to both sides created by the partnership—advantages that would be otherwise difficult to obtain (Sullivan et al., 2013). Public organizations, with responsibilities to provide necessary services in a cost-effective manner, can provide an opportunity for training, research, public policy experience, and impact at levels ranging from the individual to the larger system. Academic partners who are particularly interested in applying their resources toward service delivery, community engagement, research-generated knowledge, and system change may encounter distinctive opportunities to do so in the course of such partnerships. Both an awareness of these advantages and a commitment to publicizing them can help these partnerships to run more effectively.

Know and communicate the value brought. Part of the advantage of collaboration is the financial value associated with the delivery of services by graduate students, residents, and fellows (with appropriate supervision from professional staff). There are other aspects to the "value" associated with service delivery by trainees: energy, interest, familiarity with recent developments in the field, and sophistication in communications technology, for example.

There is continuous need for training, particularly when there is turnover. Being clear and open about the mutual advantages and value of collaboration is an early step. But as the preceding chapters make clear, personnel turnover is a recurring challenge. Some individuals who are part of these collaborations will leave their positions or graduate (in the case of students), and others who are unfamiliar with the project will replace them. When the departing individuals are directly involved in project activities (e.g., line staff, trainees), then regular training sessions and ongoing supervision can help ensure that there is less slippage from changes that have resulted from the collaboration to date. Training has been cited as a "facilitating influence" for effective collaboration (Pesta et al., 2019).

When leaders change, it can be helpful to make a modified version of such training available so their replacements can become familiar with the project. Priorities for such modified training include broader considerations such as advantages, value, and effectiveness. This kind of information can also be valuable to stakeholders, such as those receiving services and those who are not immediate collaboration partners but whose work is nonetheless influenced by the partnership. For a more detailed discussion, see Chapter 8.

Continuously renew mutual trust. A good working relationship between partners is quite important in these collaborations (Rudes et al., 2014). Chapter authors often referenced the ongoing attention needed to this working relationship and the mutual trust associated with it. Particular components of the working relationship that can promote effectiveness and trust are discussed in the following three paragraphs.

Establish clear expectations about the roles and responsibilities of each individual and entity. This can be addressed throughout the collaboration. Beginning with the initial planning and contracting, it can also be clarified during the subsequent work and modified as needed during subsequent contract discussions.

Communicate effectively. Continuous and effective communication is cited as a key component of these partnerships in the broader literature (see, e.g., Nilson et al., 2014; Pesta et al., 2019; Rudes et al., 2014). One aspect of effective communication cited by a number of collaborations includes regularly scheduled meetings. Having a designated "point person" and using a distribution list for e-mailing and text messaging can also fill in gaps between meetings but may simultaneously increase the problem of information overload unless used judiciously. Busy people working their way through many e-mails or texts can be tempted to hit "delete" quickly, leaving the sender with the misleading sense that meaningful communication has occurred. The balance involves communication that is sufficiently frequent to inform but not so frequent as to overload.

Show mutual respect. Genuine respect for collaborative partners includes an awareness of others' priorities, needs, strengths, and limitations. Even though successful collaboration typically begins with an awareness of other partners' value, there are inevitably times when partners disagree. At these times in particular, *having* mutual respect is important—but *showing* mutual respect is paramount. Many problems have arisen and been addressed in the collaborations described in these chapters. But the authors consistently emphasize the importance of mutual respect in addressing ongoing problems and collaborative challenges (see, e.g., Chapters 6 and 7).

Recognize that ethical conflicts may arise due to differing positions and disciplines. Among the particular problems that might arise in this kind of collaboration are those perceived by one partner (but not the other) as raising ethical concerns. This can be affected by disciplinary differences: those trained in one discipline may see a potential problem that does not raise ethical concerns to those in other disciplines. Examples might include public statements, social media communication, and publication. Discipline-specific ethics codes (e.g., American Psychological Association, 2010) may provide a possible resolution. To the extent that they offer guidance for members of a particular discipline doing work outside their immediate field (e.g., a psychologist conducting an evaluation ordered by a judge), the discipline member may be able to use a process involving (a) notification of others of a possible ethical conflict, (b) recommendation for an alternative course of action without potential ethical ramifications for that discipline, and (c) satisfying an ethical obligation with such notification and recommendation. What should be avoided, of course, is viewing the problem as entirely defined by the parameters of a single discipline.

Compromise. These collaborations are highly successful. They have yielded enhanced opportunities and valuable services over long periods of time. But these chapters cannot be read without recognizing the importance of compromise. Authors cited numerous ongoing challenges and, in particular, would have liked more predictable and greater funding. But the period during which most of these projects have operated (late 1990s to the present) was not one in which public organizations could easily increase (or even provide) substantial funding for such collaborations. Many projects experienced flat budgets over a period of many years. Some even absorbed cuts. But all of them were able to modify their goal of stable and growing funding, revising it to successfully operate using the same (or lower) levels of funding. It is also apparent that project growth was affected by such funding limits—so it is likely that public organizations also compromised, receiving fewer services than they might have wished.

Be good team players. A sense of working together toward shared goals can powerfully influence such collaborations. Former Indiana men's basketball coach Bob Knight uses the phrase "helpside defense" to describe an approach in which all defensive players anticipate the needs of the team based on the movement of the ball, not simply the movement of the offensive player they are defending (Knight, 2020). Using this approach, when a defensive teammate has been beaten and an opposing player has a clear path to the basket, a player must *immediately* leave his man and defend the offensive player who would otherwise score. Coaching players to do this reflexively, rather than staying with their man, proved difficult. Players have a strong urge to continue to cover their man, even when this is disadvantageous for the team. But when they did learn the helpside defense approach, it strongly reinforced an underlying sense of solidarity and shared purpose. The power of this influence should not be underestimated—particularly when it can be applied to groups working together off the court.

Be creative in problem-solving. There is clearly a role for creative approaches to addressing challenges such as limited funding and systemic inertia. Good examples of such creativity are described in Chapters 5 and 6. As interest in services grows without commensurate growth in available funding, one approach involves different uses of funding that *is* available. Another involves expanding available revenue through additional sources such as grants and other contracts. When training and consultation services are delivered but some staff members in the agency are reluctant to use them, then mutually approaching a problem (*we work together* rather than *I talk and you listen*), combined with other recommendations such as mutual respect and effective communication, can enhance the effectiveness of problem-solving.

Foster partnerships at multiple levels. One recurring aspect of these partnerships involves multiple levels of collaboration. Although the tone for this approach can be set by project leaders, this does not necessarily transfer to work involving others on either the university or the agency side. Promoting such effective interactions begins with setting a certain tone, but this must be monitored through observation, feedback, supervision, and review of products. See Chapter 10 for a clear example.

Create a community of experts. Effective collaborations do not rely on single dyads. Particularly as these collaborations grew, it was valuable to expand the existing expertise using that available from others in related areas and also available from project-involved personnel with growing expertise. Every single chapter describes expanding the pool of available expertise, some of which is accomplished by involving trainees who subsequently become experts themselves. These trainees may go on to assist the collaboration on the university side; others join the agency and bring both expertise to and perspective on the particular collaboration.

Make changes gradually. Some of these collaborations involve developing a particular service that has not been provided before (see Chapters 3 and 4). Others attempt to change how a system functions and provides specific services, as described in Chapters 6 and 8. Making changes gradually seems more applicable to collaborations with system-level goals. When there is an established approach to service delivery, there will inevitably be resistance to changing that approach. Attempted change can fail for many reasons—insufficient buy-in from leadership and insufficient resources are prominent among them—but one important mistake involves moving too quickly *when the goal is to retain major aspects of the system's functioning*. Change that is gradual allows input and discussion from stakeholders and partners, pilot testing and modification, and the establishment of greater mutual trust. Change that is abrupt, externally imposed, and/or unforeseen makes it virtually impossible to build or retain a collaborative and mutually trusting working relationship.

Training

Training is a recurring aspect of these collaborative relationships, both broadly (Pesta et al., 2019) and in the specific collaborations described in earlier chapters. It includes the role of those in formal training as they contribute to the collaboration, the provision of training to agency staff to promote quality of practice, the orientation of new members of the collaboration, and the briefing of senior leadership on both the public organization and academic sides. In this section, we discuss some of the lessons on training drawn from earlier chapters.

Provide high-quality training in relevant areas with strong training personnel. However training contributes to these collaborations, it is important. Both substantive expertise and effective training style are important when providing a briefing to leaders and stakeholders, continuing education to staff members, or an orientation to new project personnel. The majority of these collaborations included training objectives from the beginning or expanded to include significant training. There should be a good fit between university partners' capacities and the public organization's needs in the area of training. But training can also serve as a foundation on which further collaboration can develop. When training was prioritized, the collaborations were likely to involve other activities as well.

Consider whether the partnership can include opening up continuing education to outside attendees to increase exposure and defray cost. This question is particularly timely in an era in which public funding to support such collaborations is not stable. A public organization that contracts with university personnel to train agency staff could also make that training available to others who are not agency employees. Through the use of technology for communicating remotely and storing training presentations, this may offer a way to increase revenue with relatively modest additional investment. Some collaborations in which training plays a major part (see, e.g., Chapters 2, 3, 5, 6, 10) offer useful examples to other university–state collaborations that have training as a prominent part.

When creating a training curriculum, survey both administration and staff to help develop a list of relevant topics. The usefulness and viability of training relevant to practice will depend on having topics relevant to the important issues confronting practicing personnel. There may be foundational training needs that can be quickly prioritized because there is general agreement that they are indicated. Other needs, however, are best addressed by identifying them through a broader survey of agency administration and staff and searching training topics presented nationally. This may mean that training materials for certain topics are developed originally—which is actually one of the potential advantages of having a collaborative partner well-positioned to develop and present training on topics of specific need. One way in which training can be made particularly useful is through incorporating case vignettes provided by front-line staff.

Provide CE credit to encourage attendance. Continuing education credit is important for attendees who are licensed in their specific disciplines. Offering CE credit does require more work, including accessing or obtaining CE provider status; handling the details of registration, document distribution, and CE documentation; and (if the training is presented in person) obtaining training space. All this would intensify the effort needed to make the training available to interested outside individuals. Even when CE training is presented only in-house, however, providing CE credit is a bonus for staff members who need it to maintain their licensure.

Work with administration to select key trainings as "mandatory." One of the questions particularly relevant to collaborative training is how to ensure that such training is delivered to identified staff. Making a training mandatory can create resentment, while offering it on an entirely voluntary basis means that some staff members probably would not obtain the training. Successful collaborations seem to have compromised by limiting mandatory training to areas deemed essential, encouraging staff to attend other training that is not mandatory, involving staff members in delivering the training, and including incentives such as CE credit and refreshments (see Chapter 6).

Have administration visibly present at the actual training during the initial years of collaboration to publicly demonstrate their commitment to and support for the training. This encompasses more than visibly supporting training, although it does help with that. But it also provides a way of clearly showing the support of senior leaders on both sides of the collaboration. It is not necessary to ask such leaders to be present for the entire duration of training. Having them appear in the beginning and perhaps provide opening remarks can demonstrate their support without making undue demands on their busy schedules.

Combine training with detailed handouts and post-presentation knowledge appraisal so attendees can apply and test their knowledge. Certainly providing handouts (whether literally or virtually) is an important aspect of training. The level of detail in such handouts should be commensurate with the duration and level of the training, with more detailed versions provided to those who will actually need such detail in practice. Documents can also be retained and used in the course of training new project staff members.

Appraising satisfaction with the training experience is a standard aspect of CE provided by various disciplines on a "fee for training" basis and should be incorporated into this kind of training for quality improvement purposes. The question of knowledge testing—the retention and application of material provided in the training—does not have an easy answer, however. Depending on the focus, some attendees may find this insulting, while others may find it challenging due to language proficiency barriers. Yet demonstrating that material was understood and could be accessed as part of future practice is sufficiently important to justify some form of post-training appraisal. This is a question to which some of the previous lessons, such as creative problem-solving, respect, and obtaining input from multiple sources, should be applied toward an appropriate solution for the collaboration.

Be prepared for some very challenging, even confrontational, feedback from participants who resent having to attend mandatory training, and always handle such responses with professionalism and strive to find respectful areas of agreement and disagreement. This lesson (see Chapter 6 for more details) points to a problem with different potential solutions. Staff members might indeed be resentful, even confrontational, about being required to attend a training. This resentment might increase if there were post-training knowledge appraisal. But anticipating such a response might incline collaborative partners to approach this somewhat differently. Offering a clear justification for the training needs, communicated by senior leaders within the agency, would be a good beginning. Having representation from various disciplines on a committee tasked with training development could decrease the perception that it is being externally imposed. Providing options for taking the training in person or online might reduce the sense of inconvenience or imposition. Selecting a time and place that is convenient for attendees rather than for presenters conveys that staff time is respected and valued.

Consider presenting with a staff member to increase the sense of shared responsibility and buy-in from other staff members. Cross-training has been cited as a facilitating influence for collaborative effectiveness (Pesta et al., 2019). Consistent with the creation of a collaborative training endeavor, it can be helpful in several respects to include one or more agency staff in presenting on various topics. It underscores the message that training material was developed through the combined efforts of various individuals. Equally important, it reflects an awareness that the application of training materials must be contextualized by the circumstances under which they are used. Nobody is better placed to understand the limitations as well as the strengths of the service-delivery environment than a staff member who actually provides these services in this setting.

This can also be helpful when presenting more concise briefings and shorter training sessions to community organizations and city officials. Many of the advantages described in the last paragraph apply again. In addition, the perception of collaboration and shared responsibility associated with the project may be strengthened—and this is important for individuals who may have a limited understanding of the collaboration and its activities.

CONSULTATION

Another major aspect of some of the collaborations is consultation, ranging from case consultation to broader system-level consultation. These lessons are discussed here.

Identify the opinions and investment of each treatment team member to minimize conflict. When case consultation is provided to treatment teams, there can be difficulties when the consultants' opinions differ substantially from those of treatment team members. While this should not be an overwhelming problem—such consultation is, after all, requested primarily when cases are complex and perhaps puzzling—there are approaches to conveying consultation opinions in a respectful and diplomatic fashion even when they reflect considerable disagreement with treatment team's views. This is an important aspect of this lesson. *Before* delivering consultation opinions, make it a point to learn about the views and perspectives of each treatment team member. At the very least, this allows the consultants to acknowledge such opinions, describe how they were considered, and discuss why they were ultimately not adopted. Disagreement need not result in substantial conflict when it is presented reasonably, with justification, and having acknowledged other possible explanations.

Produce a written report as soon as possible after case consultation. This points to the need for a timely written product. Hopefully this would also incorporate some of the components described in the previous paragraph—acknowledgment of various possible explanations and a description of how, and why, the conclusions are provided, all presented respectfully—but it is important that it be provided reasonably soon. Consultations that do not offer written documentation of the process can be less effective because they slow down the larger process of problem-solving and do not provide a documented record of that process quickly.

Assist in selecting cases that might make a difference. The process of consultation-aided decision-making is necessarily labor-intensive for all involved. Cases and questions should therefore be selected carefully to maximize the impact of consultation, both in the immediate case and perhaps more broadly.

Financial Considerations

Stress related to financing is often discussed by university partners in these collaborations and is cited broadly as a key consideration in collaborative partnerships (Pesta et al., 2019). Financing is important to agency partners as well, although this receives less attention in the preceding chapters (and perhaps should be considered more explicitly in the future by others from the perspective of agency partners). Some of the lessons drawn from these chapters on financing collaborations are discussed here.

Contracts and grants/foundations are important sources. About half of these collaborations supplemented contractual funding from the public partner with grants from federal, state, or foundation sources. For some, this kind of funding was used instead of contractual funding to provide the bulk of the operating costs (see Chapter 8) or served as one of the major reasons for the collaboration, thus creating the opportunity to pursue grants and contracts that enhanced the prospects of either the university or the public organization itself (see Chapter 9). Seeking extramural funding is an important aspect of some of these collaborations, therefore. Grants from federal agencies or foundations that prioritize public policy or target certain populations typically require both expertise and access. University–state collaborations can provide both, enhancing the appeal of either partner alone.

State budgets ebb and flow. This was one of the most commonly recurring themes among the chapters. Across collaborations in different states, involving different partners and varying priorities, we learn that none of these projects, however successful, reports that contracts relying on support from state budgets are highly stable or predictable. Many cite reductions in funding from original levels, despite also indicating that the scope and intensity of services had increased. This probably just reflects the reality of many aspects of public funding over the lifetimes of these collaborations. Those considering or beginning new collaborations should be aware that public funding is variable and that, at some point, it is likely that funding will not be available at the same level. Successful projects have coped with his challenge by supplementing sources of public funding through expanding the modalities of income generation or working more efficiently with funding that is available. For the most part, however, these successful collaborations have *not* dealt with funding challenges by reducing the scope of the services provided.

Include yearly cost-of-living (COL) adjustments in contracts as part of a long-term plan for budget stability. This was offered by one of the projects in hindsight because there had not been yearly COL adjustments provided in their budgets. Indeed, their budgets had remained flat over a number of years—except once, when it was reduced. In light of our earlier observations, we see this lesson as overly optimistic for two reasons. First, contracts are typically renewed annually, with little opportunity to negotiate beyond the upcoming year. Second, because budgeting can be affected by a variety of influences, public organizations are understandably reluctant to enter into an agreement beyond the scope of their immediate budget year. Collaborations might be advised to hope for COL adjustments, but plan for agreements that do not include them.

Carefully consider fee-setting. This is suggested by a collaboration that developed a service to the courts (psychological evaluations of justice-involved defendants; see Chapter 3) and set the initial fee quite low. They subsequently encountered demand that might have far exceeded what they could provide using only their initial resources. While it is certainly possible that the judges were so pleased by these evaluations that they would have continued to request them even at a higher cost, it also seems likely that the initial fee was set too low and the overwhelming response was market-driven. There were a number of "unknowns" in the beginning (whether judges would ask for evaluations from a university-based clinic, whether the training experience would be help control the volume of referrals).

Creativity in funding. There are many ways in which funding streams can be combined to minimize the disruption to a collaboration stemming from funding interruptions or shortfalls. Such fiscal creativity can be a facilitator as well as a barrier to successful collaboration (Pesta et al., 2019). Chapter 5 provides a good discussion of the importance of funding creativity (still within the bounds of appropriate use of public funding, extramural grants, and foundations, of course). Their discussion includes examples such as blended and braided funding. Other chapters (see Chapters 3 and 10, for example) cite the use of grant overhead funds and other approaches to bridging shortfalls.

Educate university grants staff on the difference between research for federal grants and community service for state/local grants. Universities typically have personnel who are charged with assisting in seeking and managing extramural funding. Depending on the degree of specialization within these personnel, they may be familiar with contracts such as those discussed in this book. But such contracts are less frequently sought and obtained than extramural grants, so even university personnel who are quite familiar with the parameters of grant seeking and management may be less familiar with contracts between the university and public organizations. When university staff seek to apply federal grant standards to state contracts, for example, there is potential misunderstanding about the applicable rate of requested indirect costs. The higher university rate that is used with federal grants, if applied to a state contract, could quickly make the total cost of the contract prohibitive for the public organization partner. University personnel, including department heads, deans, and provosts as well as grant staff, should be aware of these considerations.

Personnel

Stable leadership provides continuity. We did not encounter collaborations in which there was long-standing leadership by a single individual or small group on the public organization side and greater turnover on the academic side. These may exist, of course, as the present sampling of successful projects is not necessarily representative of the broader population of such collaborations. The pattern we did see among the collaborations described in these chapters, however, involved a single leader or small group on the academic side, with greater turnover in leadership within the public organization. We conclude that stable leadership is important, and many of the other lessons in this chapter are more easily applied by someone who remains interested in the area and has worked in it for a period of time. All of these chapters reflect collaborations of multiyear durations. The best example of a very long-standing collaboration with a single leader over the years is provided in Chapter 2, involving the University of Virginia's Institute of Law, Psychiatry, and Public Policy led by Professor Richard Bonnie.

There is value in embedding trainees. One distinctive aspect of universities is their involvement in training those who will be the future leaders, shapers of public policy, practitioners of behavioral health, and researchers of applied scientific questions. The opportunity for such individuals to have the experience of working on projects described in these chapters can add extraordinary value to their training. Yet trainees may contribute as much as they receive. In every collaboration described in the preceding chapters, there was a prominent role for trainees. Indeed, without such trainees, collaborations are likely to be far more limited in scope. When provided with appropriate resources, models, and supervision, therefore, trainees bring very distinctive value to these collaborations.

Have appropriate supervisory resources. This largely positive appraisal of trainee contributions is contingent, however, on the availability of proper oversight. This appears in various forms. When trainees work with established professionals in an agency, these trainees can see both what the work comprises and how professionals in the field approach it. Formal supervision promotes trainee learning. For some trainees, it also allows them to satisfy experience requirements that are needed in applying for internships, residencies, fellowships, and first jobs. In some states, such supervised experience can also satisfy aspects of licensure requirements. This kind of modeling and supervision plays a large part in adding value to trainees' experience as part of such collaborations.

Key stakeholders have limited availability. For some of these projects, the senior leadership on both sides is a fairly small group of individuals. For others (see Chapter 8, for example), there is a broader array of stakeholders. Even stakeholders who value the collaboration's work, however, are likely to be less available for meetings and other time-consuming activities than are project personnel. Compensating for such limited availability through concise written products, regular brief updates, and the use of remote technology to make contact more convenient can help balance the importance of stakeholder participation against the reality that many stakeholders will often be unavailable.

Research

Finally, there are collaborations in which the mutual pursuit of research is among the goals. Not surprisingly, research that is oriented toward advancing knowledge of importance to a public organization is more appealing to agency partners. This section addresses three of the lessons drawn from the collaborations that did pursue research activities together.

Maintain archival data. Data of various kinds are gathered in the course of clinical and public policy projects for different purposes. They can inform decision-making about resources and services and appraisals of the effectiveness of staff work and client progress. They can offer information about the impact and cost-effectiveness of innovations. There are, in short, a variety of reasons for collecting accurate data and using them to guide policy and practice.

Preserving such data archivally can also facilitate research on clinical practice and public policy. Such archival data cannot, of course, simply be adapted for scientific use and published or presented. Archival datasets must be approved for research use by an institutional review board (IRB) or research approval committee before they can be used for this purpose. But maintaining data archivally while using them to improve policy and practice can also make it possible to eventually use such data for scientific purposes—if that is of interest to both collaborative parties *and* approved by the appropriate IRB.

Clarify the IRB approval process. The procedure described in the previous paragraph is somewhat different from that used when projects obtain data intended for both clinical and research purposes (see Chapter 6, for example). When leaders anticipate that data will be used for both purposes, then the entire procedure should be approved in advance by the IRB. This approval process may be more complex when there is more than one IRB with possible jurisdiction. A university will have an IRB; there may be an IRB for a city or state as well. Determining which IRB will have primary jurisdiction and which will conduct a secondary review is an important aspect of collaborative research.

Clarify the informed consent process. An IRB review of proposed research, defined as any activity that is intended to advance knowledge and be published or presented as such, can be more complex when the activity is also a service from which a participant may derive a clinical benefit. An IRB's review and advance approval of such a project would consider the process by which investigators obtain the informed consent of participants. This can be further complicated when the proposed research and service is conducted with "vulnerable populations," such as those who are justice-involved or who experience severe mental illness. The question of how informed consent is obtained must include how the proposed participant understands the risks and benefits and whether they choose (without being coerced) to participate. This is a necessary aspect of research done as part of such collaborations.

CONCLUSION

This volume provides an unusual opportunity to consider the collaboration between universities and public behavioral health organizations. There is a limited literature in this area, so the preceding chapters provide a distinctive look at long-standing, successful collaborations. It is likely that the need for and interest in the services provided through such collaborations is substantially greater than the number actually operating. But clearly there are key features to starting, operating, and sustaining success in this area. Reading through these chapters can guide the development of collaborative projects—particularly those that are most similar to the needs and circumstances of a proposed collaboration. This final chapter attempts to distill the lessons provided by those who have for many years engaged in the successful operation of these partnerships. To the extent that we have succeeded in documenting and analyzing the components of successful collaborations, we hope that others will find it useful—and draw encouragement for developing their own projects—to the larger good of populations we serve, the agencies that support them, and our larger society.

REFERENCES

American Psychological Association. (2010). Ethical principles of psychology and code of conduct. http://apa.org.
Burkhardt, B. C., Akins, S., Sassaman, J., Jackson, S., Elwer, K., Lanfear, C., . . . Stevens, K. (2017). University researcher and law enforcement collaboration: Lessons from a study of justice-involved persons with suspected mental illness. *International*

Journal of Offender Therapy and Comparative Criminology, 61, 508–525. https://doi. org/10.1177/0306624X15599393

Childs, K. K., & Potter, R. H. (2014). Developing and sustaining collaborative research partnerships with universities and criminal justice agencies. *Criminal Justice Studies, 27,* 245–248. https://doi.org/10.1080/1478601X.2014.947810

Knight, B. (2020). Helpside defense with Bob Knight. https://www.hoopcoach.org/ helpside-defense-with-bob-knight/

Nilson, C., Jewell, L. M., Camman, C., Appell, R., & Wormith, J. S. (2014). Community engaged scholarship: The experience of ongoing collaboration between criminal justice professionals and scholars at the University of Saskatchewan. *Criminal Justice Studies, 27,* 264–277. https://doi.org/10.1080/1478601X.2014.947809

Pesta, G. B., Blomberg, T. G., Ramos, J., & Ranson, J. A. (2019). Translational criminology: Toward best practice. *American Journal of Criminal Justice, 44,* 449–518. https://doi.org/10.1007/s12103-018-9467-1

Rudes, D. S., Viglione, J., Lerch, J., Porter, C., & Taxman, F. S. (2014). Build to sustain: Collaborative partnerships between university researchers and criminal justice practitioners. *Criminal Justice Studies, 27,* 249–263. https://doi.org/10.1080/ 1478601X.2014.947808

Rojek, J., Smith, H. P., & Alpert, G. P. (2012). The prevalence and characteristics of police practitioner–researcher partnerships. *Police Quarterly, 15,* 241–261. https://doi.org/ 10.1177/1098611112440698

Sullivan, T. P., Willie, T. C., & Fisher, B. S. (2013). Highlights and lowlights of researcher practitioner collaborations in the criminal justice system: Findings from the Researcher Practitioner Partnerships Study (RPPS). Report submitted to the U.S. Department of Justice. www.ncjrs.gov/pdffiles1/nij/grants/243914.pdf.

Worden, R. E., McLean, S. J., & Bonner, H. S. (2014). Research partners in criminal justice: Notes from Syracuse. *Criminal Justice Studies, 27,* 278–293. https://doi.org/ 10.1080/1478601X.2014.947812

For the benefit of digital users, indexed terms that span two pages (e.g., 52–53) may, on occasion, appear on only one of those pages.

Tables and figures are indicated by *t* and *f* following the page number